BE
PARA
FIT

OSPREY
PUBLISHING

Bloomsbury Publishing Plc
PO Box 883, Oxford, OX1 9PL, UK
1385 Broadway, 5th Floor, New York, NY 10018, USA
E-mail: info@ospreypublishing.com
www.ospreypublishing.com

OSPREY is a trademark of Osprey Publishing Ltd

First published in Great Britain in 2020

A catalogue record for this book is available from the British Library.

ISBN: PB 978 1 4728 3970 1; eBook 978 1 4728 3971 8; ePDF 978 1 4728 3968 8; XML 978 1 4728 3969 5

20 21 22 23 24   10 9 8 7 6 5 4 3 2 1

Originated by PDQ Digital Media Solutions, Bungay, UK
Printed and bound in India by Replika Press Private Ltd.

Illustrations by Garry Walton, © Osprey Publishing.

Photographs are acknowledged as follows: Author's collection: pp. 5, 34, 35, 139, 140, 142 (left), 145, back
cover (left), inside cover; Dennis Peeters/Wikimedia Commons: p. 24; iStock: p. 146; © IWM (H 17365): p.
155; Jeff Pachoud/AFP/Getty Images: p. 173; Julian Herbert/Getty Images: p. 21; Kai-Otto Melau/Getty
Images: p. 170; Marco Di Lauro/Getty Images: pp. 18, 138; sampics/Corbis via Getty Images: pp. 168, 169;
SUPPORT OUR PARAS (supportourparas.org): p. 176. All other photographs: Matt Timbers.

Osprey Publishing supports the Woodland Trust, the UK's leading woodland conservation charity.

To find out more about our authors and books visit **www.ospreypublishing.com**. Here you will find
extracts, author interviews, details of forthcoming events and the option to sign up for our newsletter.

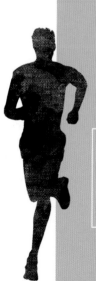

DISCLAIMER

While every effort has been made to ensure that the content of this book is as technically accurate and as
sound as possible, neither the author nor the publishers can accept responsibility for any injury or loss
sustained as a result of the use of this material. All readers should seek medical advice and consult their
doctor before commencing any exercise programme.

THE 4-WEEK FORMULA
FOR ELITE PHYSICAL FITNESS

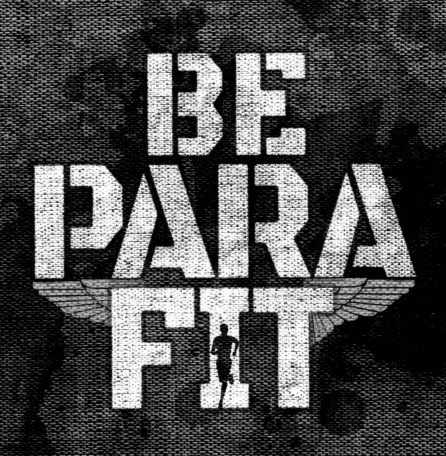

BE PARA FIT

MAJOR SAM McGRATH

FOREWORD BY LIEUTENANT GENERAL JAMES BASHALL

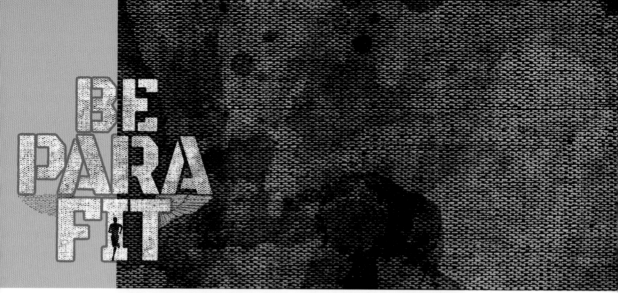

DEDICATION

For my darling wife Annie, who makes all life's experiences better and possible.

And a note for my four Warrior Princesses

Dear Eliza, Nellie, Bea and Tess,
Even if it doesn't jump out of the pages, my motivation for writing this was to impart some things to you, from the most formative period of my life. So, assuming you've inherited my lack of patience, here's the stuff I hope you will take from it.

Invest in your health. Look left and right and you'll see people readily sacrificing their health for wealth. As you grow older, you'll witness these same people willing to pay anything to reclaim even a fraction of the health they were born with. Train hard and you'll find you have more energy than those who avoid exercise, so you'll end up kicking their ass at work as well... There's not a part of my life that hasn't been enriched by fitness. Humour your old man and reach for your trainers when you find yourself tired, angry, upset, stressed or – better still – every day.

Go all in. When setting goals, a litmus test that's served me well is: does it scare me and does it excite me? If the answer is *yes*, then get to it and go all in, knowing that the quickest consume the slowest, not the biggest the smallest. As long as you learn and improve quickly, it's all up for grabs.

Pick work you believe in. It's ironic that I still define myself as a paratrooper – a life you never knew. But my first career gave me a cause I believed in as well as a contagious feeling of inevitable success that came from being shoulder to shoulder with people I loved and who were ready to take on the world. When you're driven by a calling, work dissolves and it all feels like fun.

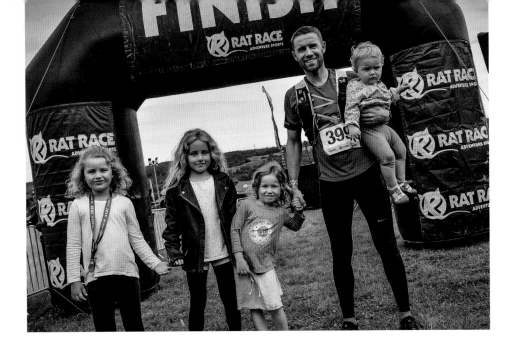

Wing it. I have never felt ready for any responsibility I found myself with – especially parenthood. My default setting has been to accept it and figure it out on the hoof. But my parachute has always been a trusted group of wise people whom I can turn to for advice, without fear of judgement. In short, if you're not feeling like an imposter in the roles you're in, you're playing it too safe – but make sure you have some good people you can turn to.

Happiness is wanting what you have. Far too many of my colleagues over the years have been too anxious about the future or discontent with the past to enjoy the present, which is all there really is. Try to live in the present, knowing that happiness is never the other side of something, no matter how prestigious, shiny or coveted. It comes from doing things you love with people you love, allocating your time and talents to help others and being grateful for what you have. The emperor is nearly always naked – but it takes courage to call it out. Choose a life of passion, not possessions.

Share it with someone you love. Everything is better shared. The hero of this story is your mum, who makes us bigger than the sum of our parts. Choose a partner who is a soulmate who challenges you to be your best self, and vice versa. The interdependence will keep you both on track, amplify every triumph and dilute every disaster.

Now tidy your bedroom!

Dad, 2019

All author royalties of the sales of this book are being donated to the charity SUPPORT OUR PARAS.

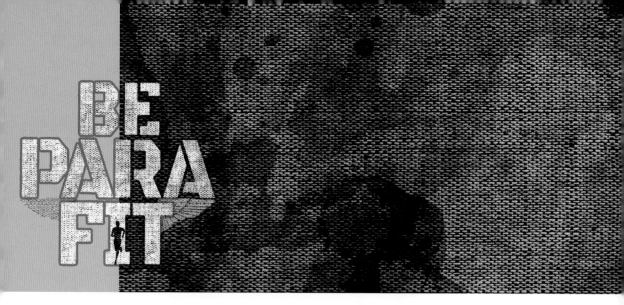

CONTENTS

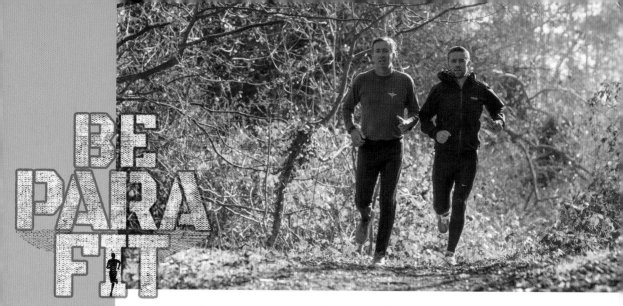

FOREWORD

I first met Sam a few weeks after the terrorist attacks of 9/11. He and I were both serving in a Parachute Battalion – 2 PARA – preparing for an emergency tour to Afghanistan. I had only returned recently to take command, and Sam was one of my young platoon commanders. It was the day of the Battalion cross country race, and Sam barely paused after introducing himself before recommending I bet the family silver on him winning. Arrogance perhaps, but in his first interaction with his commanding officer it was the essence of confidence, not least because the Parachute Regiment has exceptional physical fitness standards. Amidst all the time constraints of preparing for a hasty deployment to Kabul, he had kept himself at peak physical fitness, managing to balance this commitment alongside a myriad of pre-deployment activities. In my judgement, the concept of balance is one of life's golden threads. Those I love and admire the most seem to achieve all their goals without sacrificing health and relationships along the way. The key to this success – the underpinning key criteria – is without doubt fitness. And over the past 18 years Sam has kept himself very fit. But he is now also the father to four beautiful daughters, and happily married to his lovely wife Annie; and he has made a highly successful transition from soldier to banker. Yet through it all he has retained the same high levels of fitness I witnessed in 2001. We have continued to keep in touch since he left the army, and I have watched with growing admiration as he has achieved considerable professional success and yet still retained an incredible level of fitness alongside his growing domestic responsibilities as a husband and father.

From my perspective, after more than 30 years in the Parachute Regiment, and having served on operations and deployments across the globe, physical fitness is a quality prized above all others. Being fit is at the heart of our military selection; and it underpins the warrior mentality which is so important to success on operations. The best men and women I served alongside managed to sustain high levels of fitness to match their exceptional professional competence. But fitness doesn't end on the battlefield. As Sam shows us in this book, fitness is a part of everybody's everyday life; and total fitness which incorporates professional endeavour and strong family values is the key to successful living. Keeping fit and applying a systematic approach to training, whilst retaining a balance between work and family is the key to effectiveness both in the military and in life.

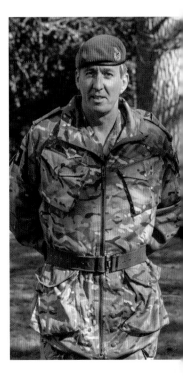

The Parachute Regiment is an organisation which relies on the individual to be physically fit, technically competent and able to function under duress. We require the total commitment of our personnel; but we also require our soldiers to take responsibility for their life and health requirements. This balance is facilitated through a mixture of military training, fitness training, sport, adventurous training, family life and social occasions; all of which provides choice and allows individuals to take ownership of their lives. Sam's book draws on his experience in the regiment to bring this to life. We encourage soldiers and officers to invest in their own fitness, but we also recognise that success requires the right mental as well as physical approach. You have to create the right training environment. Whilst the outcome is fitness focused, the building blocks are stability, determination and balance. In this book, Sam has taken the Parachute Regiment's approach to garnering success, and shown how our approach to developing the building blocks of fitness and balance can be used to develop oneself outside the military environment. The formula works for us, could it work for you?

And, in case you might still be wondering, Sam did win the race – by some margin!

Lieutenant General
James Bashall

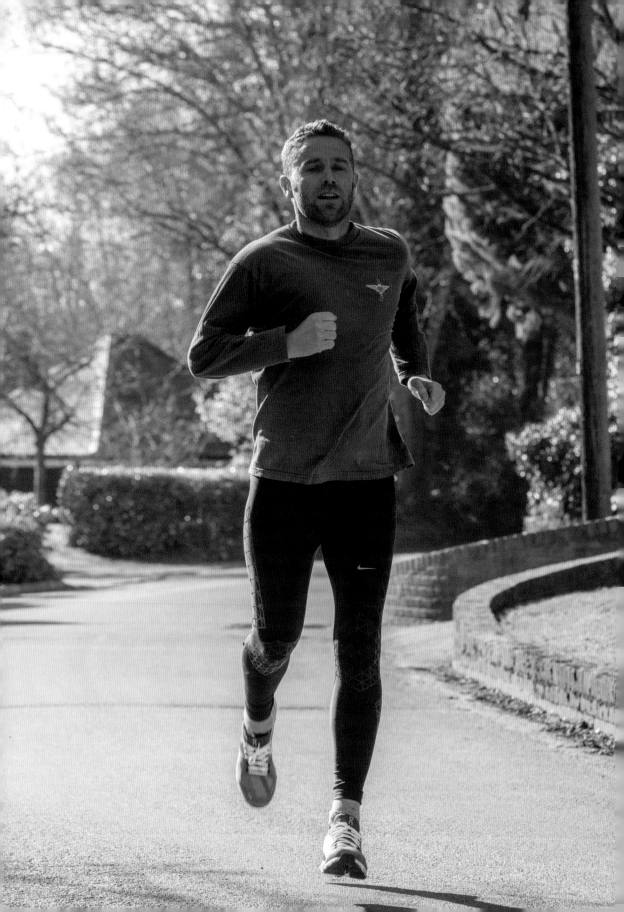

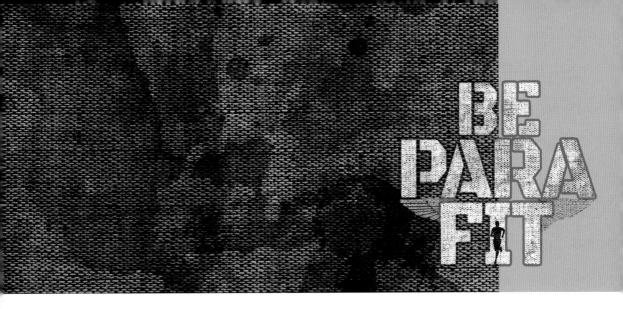

INTRODUCTION:
THE PARATROOPER SPIRIT

Over half my life ago, aged just 19, I completed selection for the elite Parachute Regiment. Of all the events that have punctuated my adulthood so far, it remains the most transformative.

Formed in the storms of war, the Parachute Regiment quickly became Winston Churchill's spearhead unit for the most dangerous and difficult military operations. Since its inception, the regiment's selection has been honed to forge the optimism, grit and self-reliance necessary to thrive in hardship and uncertainty. While parachuting may qualify as the most dramatic entrance to any battle, the regiment's ultimate success hinges on the paratrooper spirit: a tribe who together are willing to charge at hell armed only with a pail of water. What distinguishes paratroopers is their mindset, epitomized best by the Parachute Regiment maxim: *Utrinque Paratus* – 'Ready for Anything!'

LEFT 'I prefer my smock to my suit every day of the week, but I've never liked shaving' Major Sam McGrath

MY STORY

During paratrooper selection, like all other students, I was forced to weather a myriad of mental and physical storms, to push through a mounting desire to give up. But the sense of community, identity and purpose I felt was overwhelming and it was this that fuelled me through it. Being surrounded by a group of people all striving to be the best possible version of themselves and selfless in their support for one another was intoxicating and left me in no doubt that I'd made the right career choice. Something I first heard on paratrooper selection has become a mantra in every domain of my life ever since: **When you're at your lowest ebb and everything is spent, there's always at least 20% left in the tank.**

Ten years after passing the course I was selected to command it. I'd spent the best part of the intervening decade leading paratroopers on multiple tours of Iraq and Afghanistan. I was the fittest officer of my peer group and relished the opportunity to help select and shape the next generation of PARAs. Fast forward to the present, and I'm now fully immersed in the corporate world with a challenging, all-consuming role, but despite my change in environment the through line remains a rigorous fitness regime based on paratrooper training principles.

From the battlefield to the boardroom, the grit hewn on paratrooper selection has been a gift that's kept on giving. I've spent the last decade scaling the corporate ladder, raising four girls and competing at the cusp of my peer group in ultra-marathons. How do you find time, you may ask? When you decide to make fitness one of the bedrocks of your life, there's **always** time and you'll have a low tolerance for your own excuses and apologies. Training can and should be simple. Building training discipline comes quickly through purposeful practice and perseverance. While the approach I use in this book is based on paratrooper selection, the good news is you don't need to pass selection to benefit from its formula.

WHO THIS BOOK IS FOR

What separates this book from other fitness books has been weathered in my personal experience. As a former Parachute Regiment commander and Pegasus (P) Company instructor, I intimately understand motivation and the pressure of performing in the military arena. As managing director in a FTSE 100 company, husband and father of four young children, competing at the pinnacle of amateur ultra-marathon running, I've learnt how to train efficiently and effectively so it complements rather than competes with my family and work commitments. Inspired by the training and selection course I once ran, in this book I will guide you to achieve your physical fitness goals, whatever they are.

- For those looking for an antidote to an increasingly complex and sedentary work and family life: I'll help you pick the fruit of a process that's been harvested for over 75 years by the Parachute Regiment to equip people to thrive in the most challenging environments.

- For those at the start of the journey seeking to join the PARAs or similar elite military unit: I'll shine a torch and guide you on your path to what will be a formative and exhilarating period of your life.

Throughout all of the sections I'll pass on the approach I have adopted today to maintain a paratrooper standard alongside juggling multiple competing personal and professional commitments *and* being twice the age I was when I was in P Company. I will lean heavily on stories and personal accounts to illustrate and embed my approach. I will also flag the key psychological and military concepts that underpin its effectiveness, because I believe it's far easier to truly commit to something when you also understand why it works.

MY APPROACH TO FITNESS

I have distilled the systematic approach at the core of physical transformation into a model that I call the **Paratrooper Pyramid** (see Chapter 2). In essence, elite performance is founded on a firm base of **sleep**, **nutrition** and **mobility**. We will target each independently so they drive you towards, rather than drag you away from, achieving your goals. Our fitness sessions will centre on the same functional movement patterns and the endurance training used during paratrooper selection.

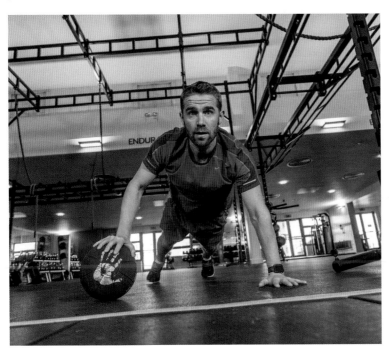

By focusing on a fixed number of functional movements and endurance activities through a four-week repeating pattern training programme, you will be able to master each pattern and focus on intensity and performance instead of perfecting a new skill. We will be striving for hundreds of marginal gains – progress which constantly compounds and multiplies – not necessarily perfection. By using benchmarks like heart rate, resistance and your most recent max repetitions you will be able to moderate intensity, so the programme evolves as your fitness improves. The effectiveness of this approach is grounded in its simplicity and its proven track record of success with the PARAs. It will also stave off injury and conserve your mental bandwidth so you're able to give your all in every single training session – and then some more...

A significant proportion of this book is devoted to efficiency. Striving for 80% of the results from 20% of the effort is as compelling as it is sensible, but be warned – there are pitfalls ahead if you apply this too rigorously in the pursuit of fitness. Read the headline of any trending fitness post and it will betray a mindset that is ultimately self-defeating. A methodology focused on losing 10kg in a month places the **symptom** (the waistline) ahead of the **system** (the lifestyle) that created it. Victims of these types of diets and fitness programmes often achieve remarkable results, only to be back in their old jeans a year later, and feeling worse for the experience. A symptom-based approach may be an extremely efficient way of changing your state quickly, but anything framed as a temporary hardship is built on shaky ground and is doomed in the long run. I am challenging you to systematically **overhaul your entire lifestyle** so you are able to deploy all of your mental and physical resources in a sustainable way.

Crossing the finish line on a bold goal, whether completing a marathon or joining the Parachute Regiment, could be the realization of consistent hard work over months or even years, but it's the hard work which makes the moment significant – not the finish line. I have far fonder memories of the mental battles fought overcoming the various hardships of Parachute Regiment selection, than in being awarded my maroon beret. It's in those moments of dealing with adversity that you achieve personal triumphs, not when they're acknowledged. The ultimate prize of paratrooper fitness is developing a mindset that's **ready for anything**.

While I may have chosen to gift the proceeds from this book to my second family, the Parachute Regiment, there's another reward I seek. When you've finished reading and integrated the relevant parts into your life, pick a goal that terrifies you and go all in. Then, when it's done, drop me a note and tell me about the journey. But nothing will prick my interest more than what you'll be doing **next** to feed your fire... *Utrinque Paratus!*

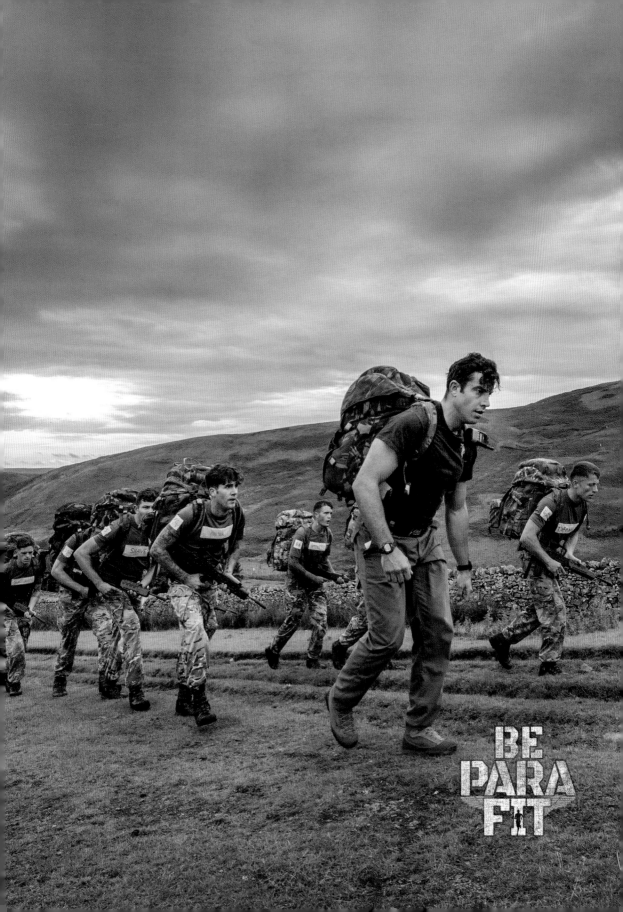

BE
PARA
FIT

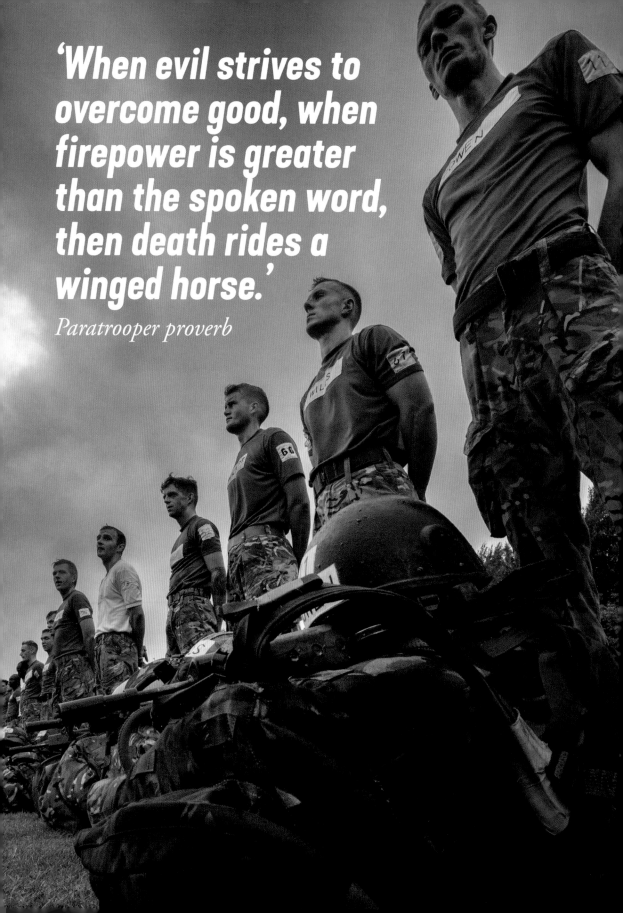

'When evil strives to overcome good, when firepower is greater than the spoken word, then death rides a winged horse.'

Paratrooper proverb

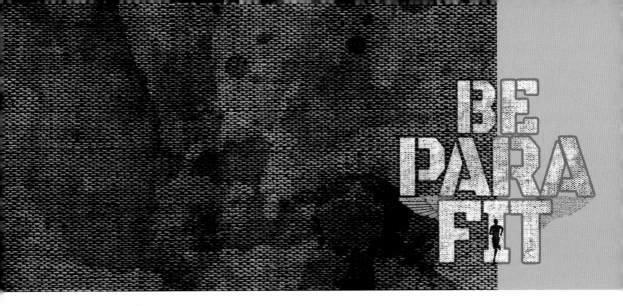

CHAPTER 1

PARATROOPERS :
THE ULTIMATE
WARRIORS

Military parachuting remains among the most difficult and important military tasks undertaken today. Parachute operations use shock tactics to achieve a swift victory. Although mass-scale drops are rare, parachute insertions remain commonplace in discrete Special Forces missions. The ability to project force rapidly and decisively is an essential tool of defence and diplomacy. Paratroopers are the ultimate warriors within any modern armed forces.

RAPID DEPLOYMENT

Paratroopers, unlike conventional soldiers, must be capable of overcoming a superior number of enemy troops armed only with the equipment they carry on their backs. Resupply is often only available by air, typically at least 48 hours after insertion due to the threat posed by enemy aircraft. In order to maximize the availability of equipment and ammunition, each paratrooper is loaded to the capacity of their parachute; their rucksacks often weigh more than they do.

Uncertainty and anxiety surround every aspect of a parachute operation. Planned in secret, each operation starts with weeks of exhaustive planning and rehearsal, frequently based on scant intelligence. Air insertions on C-130

Hercules or C-17 military transporter aircraft are long and uncomfortable. Low-level flying and hot, stuffy conditions guarantee that no one sleeps and almost everyone is sick; these conditions could have been purposely designed to degrade the passengers. By the time paratroopers have reached their destination, the fear of jumping is quickly overcome by a desire to simply get out of the flying hellhole.

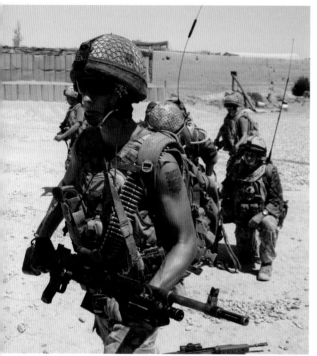 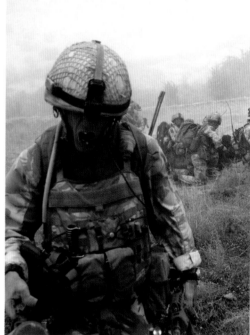

OFFENSIVE SPIRIT

For large parachute insertions, Drop Zones (DZ) are selected roughly 10 miles away from enemy objectives, a distance chosen to balance surprise with the need to avoid enemy air defences, as the PARAs are most vulnerable when jumping. The DZ is a scene of utter confusion. Terrain, weather and the enemy almost certainly guarantee that paratroopers either don't reach the DZ or land in the wrong place. The chaos of the DZ demands ad hoc planning and regrouping at every level. Soldiers and resources must be continually reallocated in accordance with changing priorities, often in the face of enemy fire.

From the DZ the paratroopers conduct a Tactical Advance to Battle (TAB). The TAB is normally a 10-mile forced march, the aim of which is to deliver the paratroopers and all their kit to their objective in under two hours, before the enemy has had time to prepare its defence. What follows is a fight for survival.

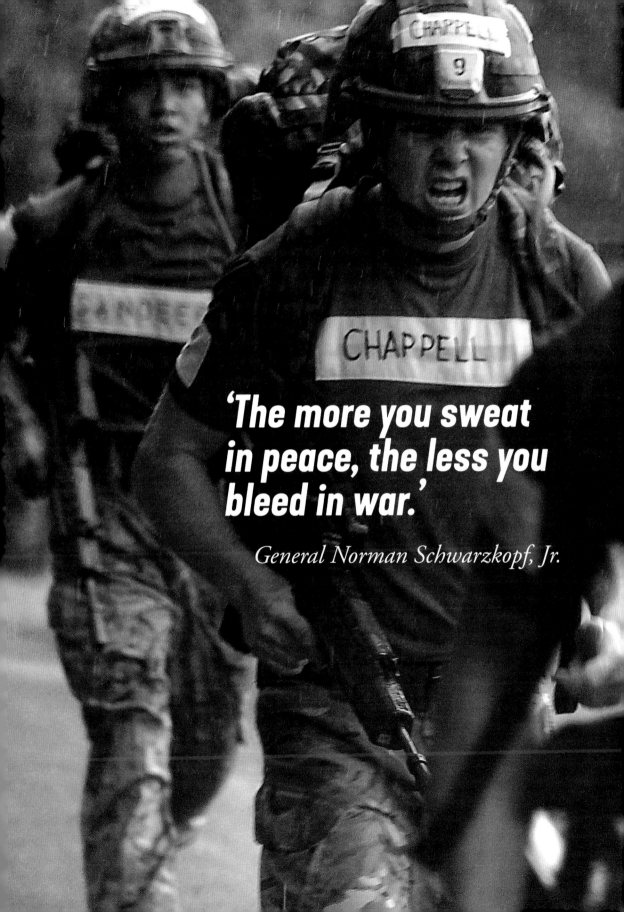

'The more you sweat in peace, the less you bleed in war.'

General Norman Schwarzkopf, Jr.

THE WILL TO WIN

For paratroopers, fitness is not an end in itself. It is a necessity to cope with the unique demands of the role. However, fitness only captures a small part of the demands placed on paratroopers. By the time a paratrooper faces their enemy, they have had to overcome numerous mental and physical obstacles that should dilute their fighting ability: uncertainty, a tortuous flight and parachute descent, and a gruelling insertion march carrying the equivalent of their own body weight in ammunition and supplies. The physical and psychological challenges of the paratroopers' role necessitate a selection and training regime with standards far in excess of those of conventional soldiers.

PARATROOPER SELECTION – PEGASUS COMPANY

Due to the unique operational role, the process of joining the Parachute Regiment is long and arduous. All soldiers, including officers, who wish to serve with airborne forces must first pass Pre-Parachute Selection. Pegasus (P) Company, the organization responsible for running this selection, consists of 12 hand-picked instructors who serve as the custodians of airborne standards. The P Company mission is:

> To test the physical fitness, determination and mental robustness, under conditions of stress, to determine whether an individual has the self-discipline and motivation required for service with Airborne Forces.

The common high standards attained by PARA recruits are fundamental to the ethos of airborne forces. By design, P Company takes students beyond their own appetite for challenge, testing their physical and mental strength, and in doing so assesses their commitment and suitability for parachute operations. The prize, for those who are successful, is the award of the coveted maroon beret and the opportunity to proceed to the Basic Parachute Course at RAF Brize Norton.

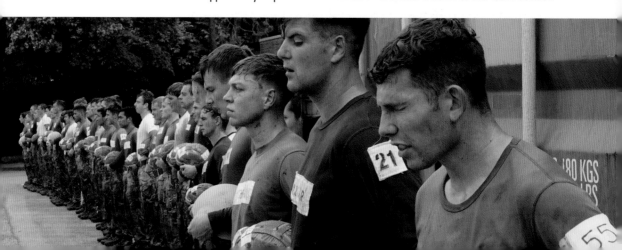

TEST WEEK

Test Week is the culmination of P Company training. Parachute Regiment recruits attempt Test Week in the latter stages of their Combined Infantry Course (CIC) in their first few months in the army. Serving soldiers are also eligible to attempt to join the PARAs, but they must pass the longer All Arms P Company course, where Test Week follows a two-and-a-half-week 'build-up' phase. Army Reservists attend a condensed four-day Pre-Parachute Selection course preceded by eight months of fitness and military training.

Test Week comprises eight separate events over a four-and-a-half-day period. Seven events are scored out of ten. However, all must pass the Trainasium event. Candidates must score a total of 45 points to pass. Points are awarded in accordance with the P Company Charter, a document that ensures the consistency of the tests and the validity of the selection. A candidate who fails to display the appropriate level of self-discipline and motivation throughout Test Week will fail the course.

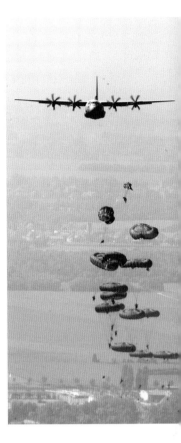

MIND OVER MATTER

The common belief that physical fitness is the only determinant of success during P Company is false. Throughout Test Week, P Company students receive no feedback on their performance. This lack of information makes the selection process much more difficult, because students spend their entire course second-guessing and worrying about whether a pass is still attainable. It is for this reason that the majority of failures during Test Week come from those voluntarily withdrawing themselves from the course. At the end of Test Week, those who pass have not only proved that they have the physical qualities of a paratrooper, but that they are able to cope with the mental stress – which on the battlefield is even more important. **This should be inspiration for your fitness journey – at times it will be lonely with little or no feedback. Like any prospective PARA, you will need to dig deep to persevere.**

Test Week starts on a Wednesday morning and finishes the following Tuesday. The tests are as follows:

10-mile march (Wednesday morning)

The 10-mile march is conducted as a squad, over undulating terrain, with each candidate carrying a Bergen (backpack) weighing 35lb (plus water) and a rifle. The march must be completed in less than one hour and 50 minutes. TA candidates have two hours. This event was the inspiration behind the PARAs' 10 charity endurance race (www.paras10.com), which I established in 2008.

Trainasium (Wednesday afternoon)

The Trainasium is a superb 'aerial confidence course' which is unique to P Company. It is used to assess and train candidates for military parachuting, specifically by testing their ability to overcome fear and carry out simple activities and instructions at heights up to 55ft.

Log race (Thursday morning)

During the log race teams of eight, carrying a 132lb log, must complete a harrowing 1.9-mile course as quickly as possible – typically within 15 minutes. This event stains each candidate's soul; to this day it remains the hardest physical challenge I have ever encountered, not least because 'coming-off' the log is considered akin to deserting your team in the midst of a crisis. The mental pressure of this rite of passage is all encompassing. When I commanded the selection course, I purposefully underplayed all other events, but amplified the pressure on the log. There is no place to hide: who remains at the end of the race is there for all to see and will be remembered by all forever.

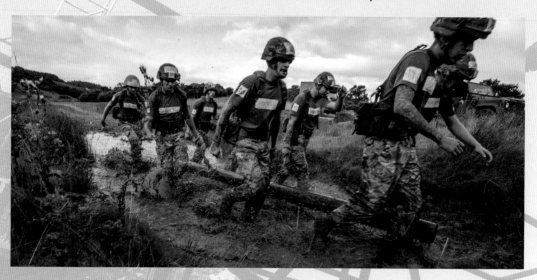

Steeplechase (Thursday afternoon)

This individual race, over a demanding 1.8-mile cross-country course, includes a number of 'water obstacles' and an assault course. Candidates must complete the event in under 19 minutes to score ten points.

2-mile march (Friday morning)

This is an individual, best-effort event, where each candidate has 18 minutes to complete an undulating 2-mile course carrying a 35lb Bergen.

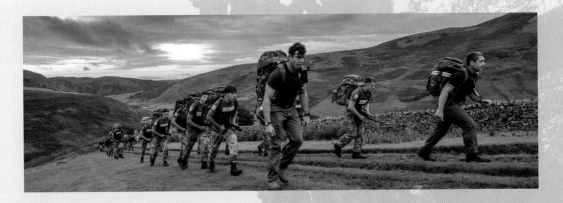

Endurance march (Monday)

Conducted as a squad, with each member carrying a 35lb Bergen, this 20-mile march over the Cheviot hills of Northumberland has to be completed in less than four hours and ten minutes.

Stretcher race (Tuesday morning)

This is the penultimate event of Test Week. Teams of 12 men take turns to carry a 175lb stretcher over a distance of 5 miles. No more than four men carry the stretcher at any given time. Participants wear webbing and carry a rifle.

Milling (Tuesday afternoon)

This 60 seconds of 'controlled physical aggression' against an opponent of similar height and weight simulates the mental stress encountered during a soldier's first contact (gun battle). The combination of neither wishing to be hurt nor perform badly among peers makes it every bit a mental battle as well as a physical one.

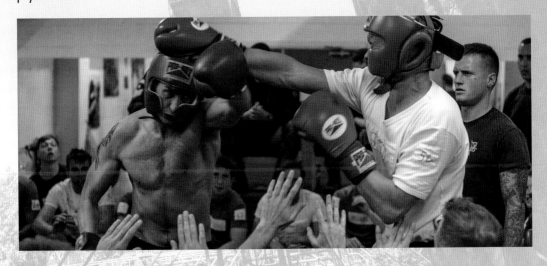

THE MERVILLE BATTERY RAID

The Normandy landings, a combined airborne and amphibious military operation that led to the liberation of France, marked a key turning point in World War II. During the planning of Operation *Overlord*, it was realized that the proximity of the selected landing points to the Merville Battery constituted a significant risk. This heavily fortified Nazi coastal artillery battery had the potential to inflict a large number of Allied casualties and even unhinge the entire operation. The battery housed four heavy artillery guns within 7ft concrete bunkers, which were protected by a mix of minefields, barbed-wire fences and 130 German soldiers. The concrete bunkers that encased the guns meant that they could only be destroyed by an unlikely direct hit from the heaviest of ordnance or by a high-risk ground assault. On 6 June 1944, the task of destroying the Merville Battery fell to 9th Battalion, the Parachute Regiment, commanded by Lieutenant Colonel Terrence Otway.

Concept of operations

The daring 9 PARA plan involved four men being inserted, ahead of the main force, to recce the target and clear paths through the surrounding perimeter and minefields. The main assault would be preceded by a barrage of 4,000lb bombs dropped from Lancaster and Halifax bombers at 0030hrs. The 650 men of 9 PARA would then have four hours from landing at their nearby drop zone to assault and secure the heavily defended position by 0500hrs, in order to prevent it from taking part in the coastal defence. Despite meticulous planning and exhaustive rehearsal, the 9 PARA attack did not go to plan. Due to a combination of navigational errors, low clouds and unforeseen problems, 9 PARA were

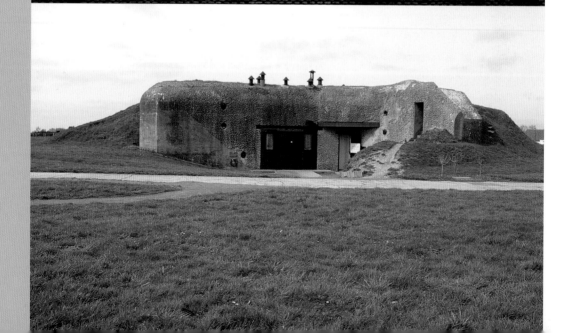

scattered up to 10 miles from their drop zone. By 0300hrs only 100 of the 650 men had assembled at the rendezvous point; most notably absent were the Land Rovers, anti-tank guns, mortars, mine detectors, medical personnel and engineers. Another critical blow was that the RAF bombers had dropped their bombs well short of the target, causing no damage to the artillery guns. However, the advance party had performed their role brilliantly, conducting a thorough reconnaissance of the target and clearing what would prove to be four vital paths through the defence perimeter and minefields.

Seizing the initiative

In true airborne spirit, Lieutenant Colonel Otway, knowing that the fate of the lives of thousands of Allied soldiers depended on 9 PARA completing its mission, redistributed his men and gave the order that the battalion (now less than one-sixth of its strength) would proceed with the men and equipment they had. Though subjected to intense enemy fire and landmine explosions, 9 PARA launched into the Nazi stronghold with the ferocity that has become synonymous with airborne forces. The Germans held all the advantages – superior numbers and equipment and the occupation of a heavily defended position. But nothing would deter 9 PARA. In the final stages of the battle, the paratroopers, who had expended all of their ammunition, were forced to engage the Nazis in hand-to-hand fighting in order to secure their objective. By 0500hrs, 9 PARA, at the cost of 65 men either dead or seriously injured, had control of the Merville Battery and had successfully prevented it from firing upon the Normandy beaches.

The 9 PARA Merville Battery raid illustrates how an approach instilled during selection and training is translated to the battlefield. Put more simply, it was a combination of daring and bloody-minded determination that enabled 9 PARA to succeed.

I believe much can be learnt from accounts such as this one. Whether battling against a fierce enemy, or against mental and physical barriers that prevent you from accomplishing the things you want to achieve, the decisive battle takes place in your mind – and to win you must believe that the rewards that come with success outweigh the cost of attaining them!

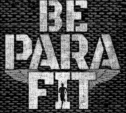
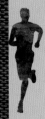

THE PSYCHOLOGY OF SELECTION

As the Merville Battery raid aptly illustrates, paratrooper missions are rife with danger and complexity. When paratroopers embark on something tough, they must lock arms and keep them locked as the pressure builds. The PARAs have delivered in adversity on countless occasions and continue to do so. Without a doubt, the crucial aspect of their success equation lies in the selection process. It instils an unparalleled strength of mind and body in the individual soldier, while at a team level forges a tribal sense of community, identity and shared purpose that time and time again is a battle winner.

THE PARATROOPER MINDSET

I believe the psychology of selection is far more than an insight into the regiment: it is a potent formula that can be transformational for achieving any **stretch goal** – a goal that cannot be achieved by minor changes or improvements but through systematic changes in all aspects of life (see below). Many qualities about the PARAs in P Company are readily visible – fit and fierce-looking soldiers wearing distinctive insignias – but I believe the real alchemy lies beneath the surface and is directly relevant to crossing the finishing line of your own audacious goals. Both are all-consuming, fully immersive experiences, but are inherently simple. The mental and physical pain you experience on the journey to achievement in each creates the conditions and stimulus for change, and with it, growth. Advancement is competency based; at each step you must develop the mental and physical patterns required to propel you to the next level. Put simply, there's no hack or instant success formula: **you have to think big, back yourself and then consistently work your ass off**.

Selection processes, like the one for P Company, exist to support operational excellence in a specialist role, not to preserve elite status. These courses not only test but build individual capability alongside commitment to 'the cause'. The process of putting volunteers through seemingly impossible tests forces them to face personal boundaries and, in doing so, proves the boundaries are false. In effect, being selected is self-fuelling, and the selection doesn't just isolate the right attitude and aptitude but creates it. The Parachute Regiment have 'P Company', The SAS have 'hills phase', the Royal Marines have the 'Commando Course' and the US Navy SEALS have 'hell week'. All create a mindset that's comfortable exploring the dark frontiers of adversity and bulldozing self-doubt.

At a team or unit level, selecting and forging the right aptitude and attitude in individual members creates an effect that's even more profound. As like-minded people are grouped together, their confidence and high professional standards skew the norm to create a high-performance culture. Mutual trust and

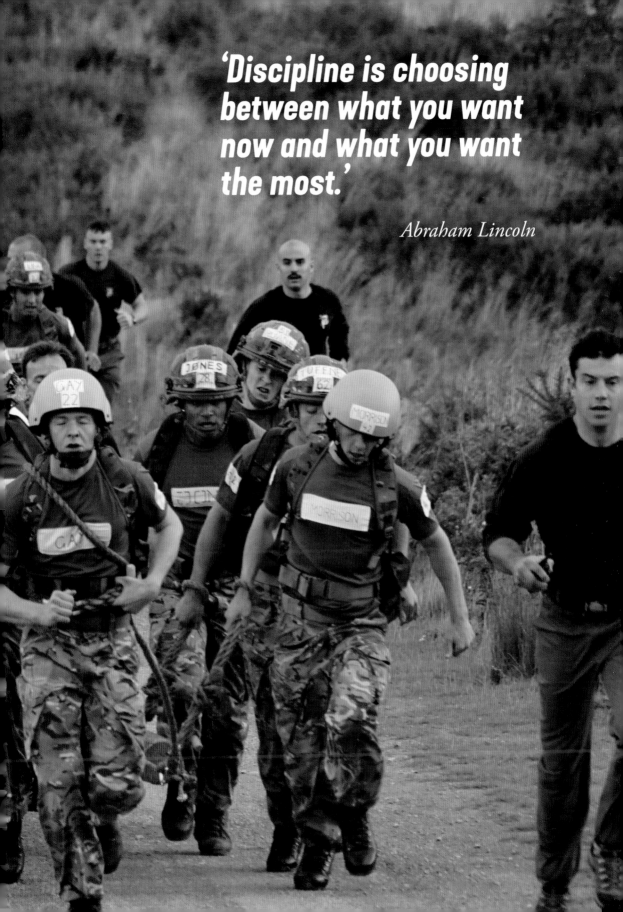

'Discipline is choosing between what you want now and what you want the most.'

Abraham Lincoln

accountability between team members is pervasive. At the same time, the veil of mystery surrounding the elite soldiers' most daunting tests and heroic feats of strength builds a reputation of military effectiveness, which intimidates those who face them in battle. And so, as confidence and fear are both contagious, the Parachute Regiment goes into battle expecting to win, having dedicated their practice to that being the only possible outcome. Their enemy, having heard about their foe's superhuman selection and professional standards, expects to fail: soon both are proven correct.

THE P COMPANY FORMULA

Paratroopers and world-class fitness athletes share three qualities: **optimism**, **self-reliance** and **grit**. There's no shortcut to acquiring these qualities. The hardship they've overcome by pushing through progressively more difficult challenges propels them to a higher level of performance built on a better understanding of what they're capable of. It is through enduring adversity that you too can create the mental patterns of optimism, self-reliance and grit that will enable you to thrive in the most challenging arenas. Here's how it works.

Optimism

To embark on something that both scares and excites requires and develops optimism. Even considering tackling P Company, a marathon or an ultra-marathon demands questions like: What pain and discomfort am I prepared to struggle through, and what am I willing to sacrifice to achieve it? Balancing the fear and risk of public failure against the perceived value of achieving it weighs heavy. The power of publicly committing to a goal with such inherent pride and jeopardy attached to it cannot be overstated. But it's optimism alone that ignites the starter pistol; how much you believe it's possible determines how much you're willing to risk and sacrifice to achieve it.

Self-reliance

Committing to a goal is the first step to achieving it. But progress is never linear, and the path is often littered with diversions and pitfalls seemingly designed to take you off track. Having committed to a goal, paratroopers must then research and develop their plan for achieving it. Anticipating and grappling with difficult questions and potential dilemmas can't be avoided. Self-reliance provides both the compass and vigilance in all decisions, prioritizing long-term success over short-term convenience. Adjusting lifestyle habits and undertaking activities that introduce anxiety and physical pain are undesirable in the short term, but ultimately are what spur progress. Those who cave into the desire to skip training

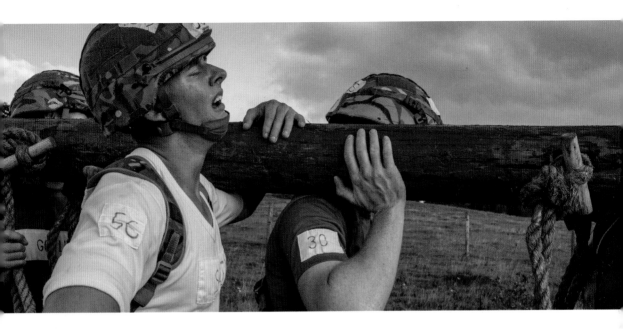

falter. Those who stay the course prevail. As the stakes rise on P Company, the challenges recruits face are both cumulative and progressive, making each milestone more difficult. At the same time, as each milestone is passed, the recruit becomes more invested and focused on their long-term goal. The successful keep their eye on the prize, while narrowing their focus to each incremental step at a time, to avoid being intimidated by the distance between them and their maroon beret.

A key aspect of self-reliance is the perception of control over personal outcomes, which is a **growth mindset**. Someone lacking this quality believes life is controlled by external factors such as fate, which they're unable to influence: this is a fixed mindset. Someone with a fixed mindset believes their abilities are innate and to succeed requires an external advantage – to cheat or find an easier challenge. In contrast, **someone with a growth mindset views failure as an opportunity from which to learn and develop**. An emotional response to failure is normal with both. But with a growth mindset, when the disappointment of a negative result passes, you can embrace the opportunity to learn and be better prepared for the next challenge instead of blaming the fairness of the test.

Aspiring paratroopers start to recognize the control they have on their physical outcomes and start building a growth mindset long before P Company commences. During Test Week students are forced to listen to themselves and learn how they react when things get tough, so they're able to replicate successful thought patterns and behaviours and eliminate the negative. There are many

'Courage isn't having the strength to go – it is carrying on when you don't have the strength.'

Napoleon Bonaparte

STRETCH GOALS AND INTRINSIC MOTIVATION

Elite selection courses and stretch fitness goals both develop intrinsic motivation to train in those who persevere despite the hardship.

You need to satisfy three psychological needs to develop intrinsic motivation for an activity:

- **autonomy:** the feeling you're doing the activity out of free will;
- **camaraderie:** the sense of being surrounded by like-minded people;
- **competence:** the perception of being capable and able to predict outcomes of the activity.

By design, success on a selection course meets these needs, but the psychological drive to train develops simultaneously with qualifying as a paratrooper, over a four-phase process.

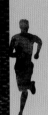

dark places on the route to winning a maroon beret or crossing the line on an adventurous fitness goal, but a growth mindset is an essential partner in navigating them and emerging stronger and better prepared for the next one.

Grit

While optimism and self-reliance are essential, they're both impotent without grit. Grit is the ability to push through adversity and to bounce back from trauma. It's a passion and perseverance for long-term goals. Its building blocks are audacity, ambition and persistence. It is also a flexibility borne out of necessity, finding comfort in a state of constant change, but even more so the ability to adapt and innovate. Performance is built on acquired strength, endurance, discipline and willpower. During P Company, paratroopers develop grit through a combination of controlled activities that incrementally add physical and mental stress.

STRETCH GOALS

An important motivating factor in the PARA fitness programme is establishing a 'stretch goal' – a long-term training objective that could all too easily be dismissed as unachievable but with the right mindset, effort and support provides the catalyst to rocket propel you forward on your fitness journey (see Chapter 6 for more on goal-setting). Stretch goals are fuelled by motivation every step of the way; without a deep well of motivation, all effort expended contemplating it is for nought. Optimism, self-reliance and grit help you navigate each challenge, but it is motivation that fires your desire to take on the goal in the first place.

There are two types of motivation: extrinsic and intrinsic. Extrinsic motivation is when you do something to receive a reward or avoid a punishment; intrinsic motivation is when you get pleasure or value from the activity itself. Developing the fitness to pass P Company starts out as an extrinsically motivated activity but over time evolves to being intrinsically motivated. So, early on the key lies in identifying the pain and pleasure points that will keep you striding forward. There needs to be a compelling why, or you'll fall flat at the first obstacle.

PHASE 1 – EXTERNAL REGULATION

External Regulation is when the activity is driven by the desire to achieve a reward or avoid punishment. Aspiring paratroopers start training long before they wear a military uniform, even when this often feels boring and lonely. The reward they're chasing is acceptance into the PARAs, while the punishment they're trying to avoid is public failure: their training is driven by the two motivating elements of pain and pleasure.

So, when you begin your first four-week training programme as outlined in this book you too will need to confront the elements of pain and pleasure. Intelligently navigating the first phase of four weeks will be the linchpin of your success. The table below illustrates the vast gains that can be made along your fitness journey, as well as the necessary 'pains' that go along with them. The 'Do Nothing' columns clearly illustrate the classic adage 'No pain, no gain!'

Journey to Being Paratrooper Fit		Do Nothing	
Pain	Pleasure	Pain	Pleasure
Risk of injury	Feeling good	Loss of self-respect	Easy
Feeling embarrassed	Health benefits	Feeling embarrassed	Can continue with current lifestyle
Don't know how	Losing weight	Unable to participate in physical activities	
Feeling discomfort	Greater self-esteem	Getting progressively less healthy	
Hard work	Gaining confidence	Risk to long-term health	
Less in common with friends	Meet new people		
Less free time	Relieving stress		

PHASE 2 – INTROJECTION

Introjection describes an unconscious psychological process in which a person adopts the behaviours and attitudes of others around them. During the time spent preparing for P Company, there are many things the future PARAs would rather do, but collectively they are working toward a common goal, which in itself fosters self-motivation to perform to their best ability. The group attitude becomes embedded in the individual, which helps to acclimatize PARAs to the necessary pain that accompanies long-term gain. The end result is the development of a strong self-reliance within all paratroopers.

At about the four-week point in your training programme, you will start feeling the benefits of your training and the regime will feel more like a habit, so despite the continuing hardship you will feel better able to choose long-term success over short-term comfort. This will make training easier.

PHASE 3 – IDENTIFICATION

By this phase, aspiring paratroopers recognize the underlying value of their training. They start to like the feeling they get from being fit and looking in better shape, which they associate with training. They're not experiencing enjoyment from training, but from its consequences. They start to identify themselves as fit and enjoy being associated with it by friends and family.

At about three months into your training regime, maybe sooner, friends and family members will start marvelling at your mental and physical mettle. This will feel great and you'll want to persevere.

PHASE 4 – INTEGRATION

By Phase 4 training is undertaken for its own enjoyment and satisfaction. Integration goes hand in hand with grit, and it is built by overcoming intimidating challenges. At some point on P Company, paratroopers connect their tremendous sense of achievement with the training that got them there. Go in any PARA unit gym and you'll witness what is almost a euphoria on the faces of people all pushing themselves to breaking point. As I know from personal experience, once you've tasted this feeling you can't imagine life without it.

I can't give you a timeline for when exactly you will experience this, nor can I provide a shortcut, but the hallmarks will be a mix of personal pride and surprise in overcoming something that once scared and excited you. From then it will feel like you're running downhill fuelled by 'the force'.

MAN VS LAKES

At the start of 2018, my wife Annie and I decided to merge a number of goals. She would complete her first ultra-marathon adventure race, and I'd do it with her; we'd also combine it with a family holiday with relatives back in the UK, which would make it possible for our girls to watch us running it. While we're both into training and racing, up until 2018 the furthest Annie had ever run was a half-marathon. As expats living in Singapore, we also lack the support network of extended family members so we usually need to take races in turn, to enable the other to look after the kids.

We picked a 50km race in the UK's Lake District called 'Man vs Lakes', with about 4,000ft of cumulative ascent. We booked our flights as well as a holiday cottage in Coniston, 1km from the finish, and invited our family to come and join us. We put a plan together, including some other races in the lead up to 'Man vs Lakes' in June. We trained hard, with some good results in our practice races in May, but after that everything went badly.

Adaptability and resilience

In the three weeks prior to the race neither of us was able to train. Annie was in the UK alone with all four of our daughters and I was barred from running while receiving physio for an injured calf. I'd meant to be in the UK weeks before the race for work, but in the end landed the morning before, just in time to attend the mandatory registration kit check. I hadn't slept on the plane the night before, and then both Annie and I got another rubbish night's sleep, trying to pacify our daughters, who were unsettled about being in a new place. We woke the morning of the race feeling tired, put off by our lack of training and perhaps just as much by the driving wind and rain we saw outside the window. Annie turned back from the half-opened curtain and in an instant left me in no doubt about what the day had in store and why I'd asked her to marry me. 'We need to do this,' she said. 'It's the first race the girls will see us do and they'll need know you don't wobble when things don't go to plan.' After a fleeting breakfast, we both jogged down to the race event area to catch the bus to take us to the start at Morecambe Bay.

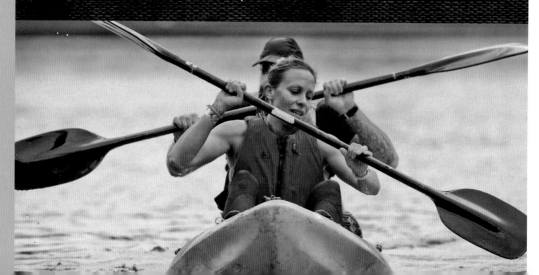

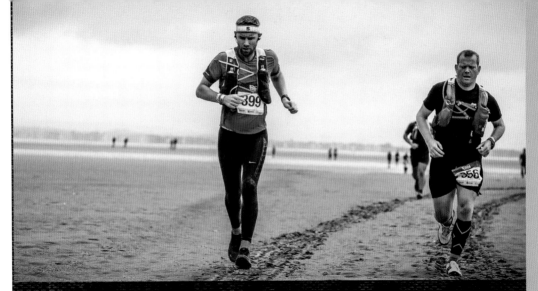

Fighting through

As soon as we left the house everything, including the weather, started to brighten up. It was great to be around fell runners. Neither of us had crossed Morecambe Bay before and the lakes were as beautiful as ever on the course. Among the 800 runners I even bumped into a colleague I had served with in 2 PARA. By the time we both reached the finish line, the weather was glorious and our kids were loving seeing their parents pushing themselves over trails, hills, and water obstacles. To top it all I came 5th and Annie was the 9th place female runner. Despite the worst preparation for any race either of us had ever entered, it turned out to a brilliant family day out, even if we all overdid the fish and chips at the finish line.

Orchestrating success

Compare this event with my time in P Company and the only thing that's materially different is the time available for training – in P Company I did not have to juggle work and parental responsibilities on top of training. The goal was no less important, no less ambitious, and the plan to realizing it no less considered. While Annie and I had endured a difficult month prior to the race, both of us had invested in our training and were mentally prepared. We surprised ourselves with what we were capable of on the day and were delighted we had followed through on making our shared goal a reality. But above all, we were proud to have demonstrated to our girls that neither a lack of time nor our varied work and family commitments were barriers that couldn't be overcome with a combination of early investments and the right mindset. We'd sealed our performance in January when we committed to it together, while momentum and mutual accountability got us to the start line.

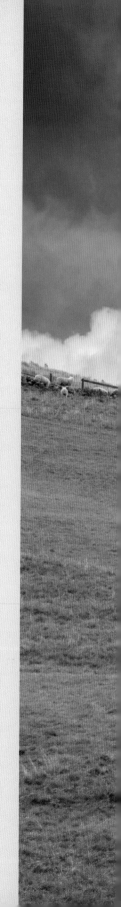

ESSENTIALS FOR STARTING YOUR FITNESS JOURNEY

Before you even break a sweat, we need to remember the three key elements to maximize your chance of success:

1. **Stretch goal.** Like P Company you need to pick a specific over-the-horizon goal that inspires you long into the future (e.g. joining the Parachute Regiment or completing your first marathon in a certain time); the more this excites and scares you, the better. This will foster **optimism**, **self-reliance** and **grit**. Whether P Company or marathon, the final result will be a mind and body that's 'ready for anything'.

2. **Sustaining discipline with pain and pleasure.** The foundation of your fitness transformation will be built on vigilance in your first 28 days. You will need to prioritize long-term success over short-term convenience. Remember: 'No pain, no gain!' This will be the best route to achieving your goals both in the short term and in the long term.

3. **Efficient execution.** The key to success will be a robust **training formula** that systematically integrates fitness into your life. You not only need to understand what's required but appreciate how and why it will work for you.

The focus of chapters 2–5 will be imparting the paratrooper training formula. In chapters 6 and 7 we'll switch focus to defining a stretch goal, including some inspirational challenges. I cannot stress enough how **the linchpin for success lies in ensuring your fitness regime complements rather than competes with family and work commitments.**

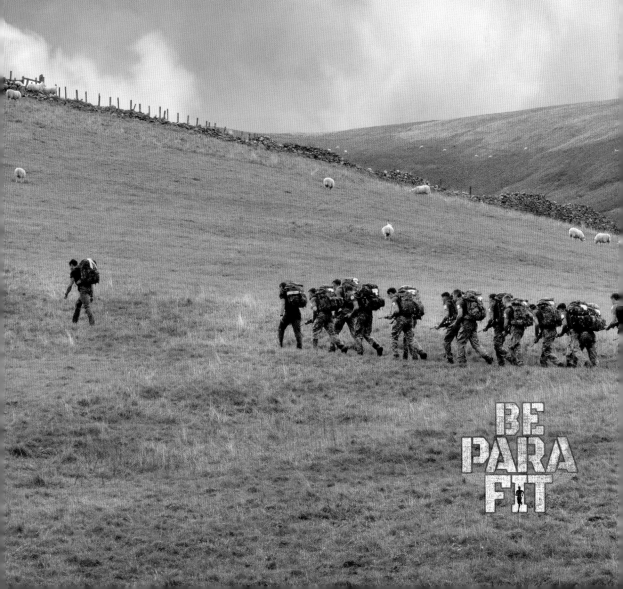

'Your comfort zone is a wonderful place, but nothing grows there.'

P Company Proverb

BE PARA FIT

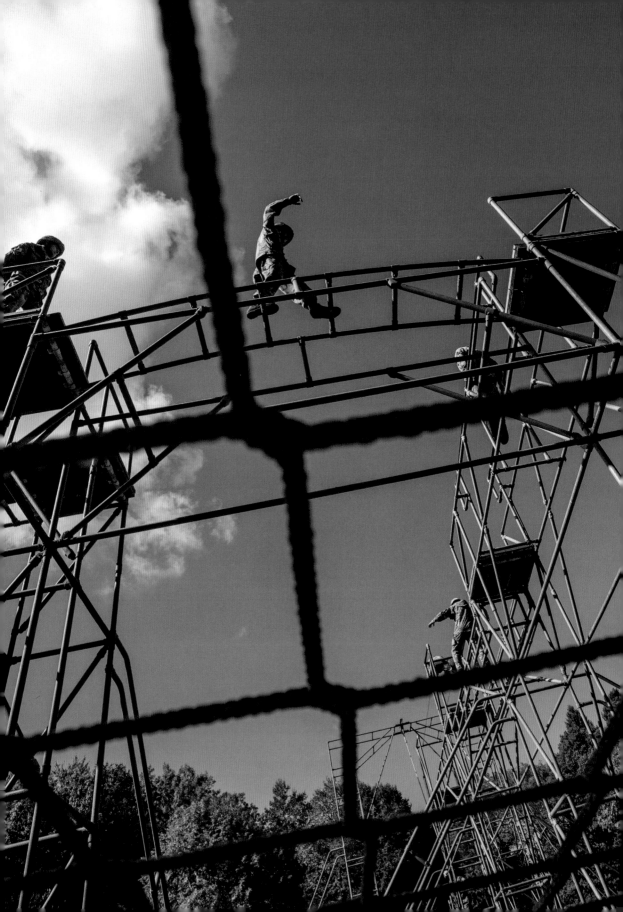

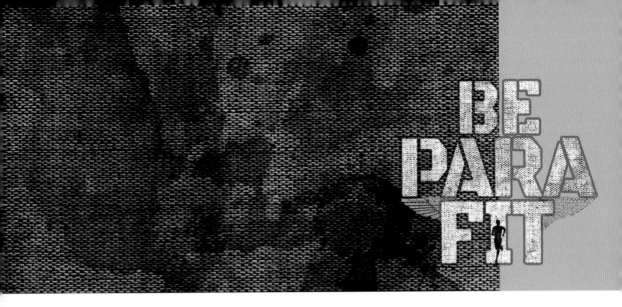

CHAPTER 2

THE PARA FOUNDATIONS OF MENTAL AND PHYSICAL FITNESS

TRAINING VS EXERCISE

I need to start with a distinction between two phrases that are often used interchangeably in a fitness context: exercise and training. Exercise is an activity done for its own sake. If done often enough and complemented with a healthy lifestyle, it will have a positive impact on your life. But let's not confuse exercise for its own sake with a purposeful march towards a long-term stretch-goal objective. By contrast, training describes the process, not just the constituent sessions of the process. Training takes time, instruction, dedication and, ultimately, a goal. Building an effective training plan is about focusing on maximizing each component for optimal performance.

THE BENEFITS OF PHYSICAL TRAINING

A weekly training programme comprising 2x aerobic activities and 2x strength sessions has been linked to the following health benefits, from extensive scientific research:

Improves cardio function. Training optimizes the heart's function and overall efficiency. A strong heart provides more oxygen, nutrients and energy to your body throughout the day. Training increases High-Density Lipoprotein (HDL) (good cholesterol), alongside decreasing harmful Low-Density Lipoprotein (LDL) (bad cholesterol) and reducing blood pressure.

Strengthens bones. Weight-bearing activities, such as running or strength and conditioning training (like circuit training), increase bone density and support muscular development.

Improves mood. Training releases endorphins, hormones that produce a feeling of euphoria. Exercising outdoors supports the creation of vitamin D, which is linked to cognitive function, while its absence is associated with mood swings and depression.

Improves self-esteem. The cocktail of endorphins and sense of accomplishment derived from exercise improves feelings of self-worth. The physical gains of exercise (reduced body fat, larger muscles, general toning) multiply this effect.

Relieves stress and anxiety. Training releases norepinephrine, a hormone that regulates and reduces your stress, the perfect antidote to a cortisol-fueled professional life.

Improves sleep quality. Exercise helps anchor the circadian rhythm, your body's natural clock, which tells it when it's time to go to sleep and wake up. Exercise is most effective first thing in the morning, when accompanied by daylight. Always allow 90 minutes after exercise before going to bed to allow endorphin levels to subside.

Improves memory and learning. Aligned to sleep, exercise promotes neurogenesis, the creating of new synapses which support memory and learning.

Increases metabolism. Exercise not only burns calories while training, but the adaptation process created in the body following activity spurs muscle growth, which burns calories while sleeping.

Optimizes digestion. Exercise relieves the symptoms of conditions such as constipation, bowel disorders and liver disease. It reduces the risks of some colon cancers and stomach ulcers. The mediating effect of exercise on stress, a risk factor in digestive disorders, also supports broader gut health.

Moderates appetite. Exercise acts as both an appetite suppressant and a key motivator in optimizing your approach to nutrition as a means of enhancing the effectiveness of your training programme.

Reduces risk of infection. Exercise is a key ally in reducing the risk of developing Type 2 diabetes, strokes, and some forms of cancer.

SYSTEMIZING TRAINING

During Parachute Regiment training all activity is geared towards a particular performance outcome – competence across a set of specific battle skills and reaching the standard of P Company. All training is structured: no assumption is overlooked, no training session is wasted, and nothing is included merely to fill time. Raw military recruits are taught how to stand, march, crawl and even how to wash. Parades are used to instil discipline to words of command, as well as to correct issues with body posture. Drills are used to implant instinctive coordinated responses to potential sources of danger, both planned (such as parachuting) and unplanned (such as reacting to an ambush). Efficiency and effectiveness are merely a collage of set pieces, individually and collectively honed in training, and refined constantly in response to failure.

Whether your goal is acquiring paratrooper fitness or joining the Parachute Regiment, the quickest and surest route to victory is to follow a training plan that simultaneously invests in sleep, nutrition and mobility alongside strength and aerobic endurance activities. If executed as intended, each day will build on and complement the previous. The three essentials of sleep, nutrition and mobility must first be satisfied before you can reap any of the physical benefits of training. I will discuss each of these key aspects in more detail below.

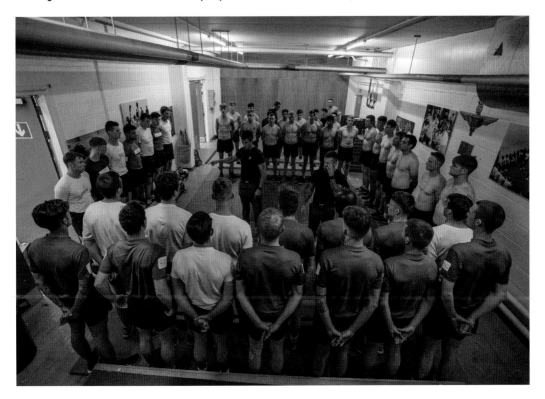

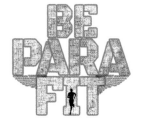

THE PARATROOPER PYRAMID

The Paratrooper Pyramid represents the relative importance of the components of optimum health and performance. Achieving paratrooper fitness requires focused training and purposeful practice. But any compromises made to sleep, nutrition and mobility will be a net drag on your progress of at least 4:1. Put another way, someone who eats, drinks and sleeps intelligently and complements this with a blend of two to three uncoordinated exercise sessions will achieve far more than someone who invest 16 hours into a well-refined training regime and ignores sleep, nutrition, mobility and hydration.

Although the human body has remained virtually unchanged for 200,000 years, the lives we now lead could not be more different than those of our ancestors. A fit human, by definition, represents an optimal expression of our evolutionary makeup. We were designed to run, hunt, live off the land, fight off predators – to *move*. Yet, we find ourselves in a world that predisposes us to too much sitting, sugar and

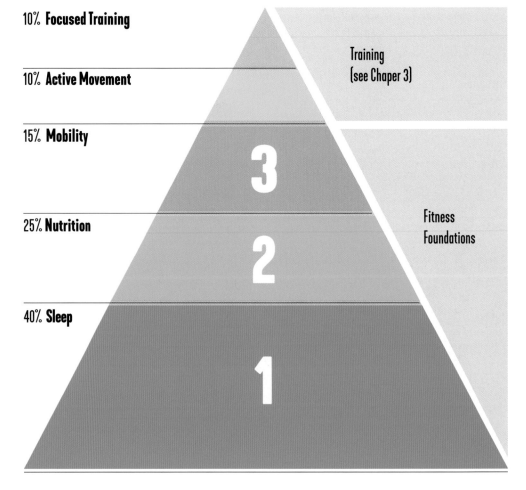

10% **Focused Training**

10% **Active Movement**

15% **Mobility**

25% **Nutrition**

40% **Sleep**

Training
(see Chaper 3)

Fitness
Foundations

3

2

1

screen time, which as a mode of living is like kryptonite to life itself. Regaining control of our ancestral vitality demands structure and discipline: to move more, consume less and go to bed earlier than you might want to.

At 40, with a demanding job, four kids, a time-consuming writing hobby and six hours to train a week, my VO2 Max is 72, the average of a male Olympic athlete in their twenties. Without a significant change of focus I will never win anything big, but 8th place was my worst result across four ultra-marathons in which I competed last year and I feel great for all 168 hours in a week. Six hours a week of focused training activity is what you need to replicate and hopefully exceed this, but let's not attempt to rearrange the roof tiles before we've laid the foundations. The **three essential building blocks of sleep, nutrition and mobility** must be satisfied first.

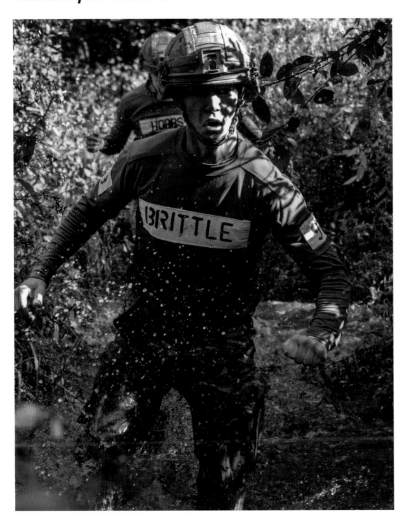

VO2 MAX – SCIENTIFIC MEASURE OF FITNESS

VO2 Max is the predominant means of measuring aerobic fitness. It is expressed as 'relative rate of oxygen processing capacity (ml per kg of body mass)', varies greatly between individuals and can be improved with training. Also referred to as 'maximal aerobic capacity', VO2 Max reflects the cardio-respiratory fitness of an individual and endurance capacity during prolonged exercise.

VO2 Max improves with training and can be doubled in some individuals. Research suggests that VO2 Max is 50% genetic and 50% influenced by training and lifestyle. Aerobic training improves VO2 Max through training adaptation, but is best optimized using a training programme that includes at least a weekly interval training session. Research has identified that 2- to 5-minute efforts at 3km race pace is ideal for improving VO2 Max.

Accurately measuring VO2 Max involves exceeding the aerobic capacity of an athlete, normally on either a treadmill or cycle ergometer, using a maximal and progressive test. Throughout the test, the athlete's aerobic ventilation is measured, including the composition of oxygen and carbon dioxide inhaled and exhaled. VO2 Max is reached when oxygen consumption no longer increases, despite an increase in workload. The test is used widely by amateur athletes and professionals to measure fitness and progress. Sports labs in most major cities offer the test for around £50 GBP. The test takes 30 minutes, is extremely difficult and should only be undertaken in good physical health. Many approximations exist, including applications within most heart rate (HR) and global positioning system (GPS) devices. These approximations use an algorithm to triangulate personal data (height, weight, age, gender) with load data (HR and speed). The best algorithms are 95% accurate compared with laboratory testing.

Key points:
- universal scientific measure of aerobic fitness;
- extremely difficult test as it requires maximal performance output;
- proxy tests widely available, cheap and 95% accurate;
- improved using mix of aerobic and interval training.

Female VO2 Max Levels

Age	Very Poor	Poor	Fair	Good	Excellent	Superior
13–19	<25.0	25.0–30.9	31.0–34.9	35.0–38.9	39.0–41.9	>41.9
20–29	<23.6	23.6–28.9	29.0–32.9	33.0–36.9	37.0–41.0	>41.0
30–39	<22.8	22.8–26.9	27.0–31.4	31.5–35.6	35.7–40.0	>40.0
40–49	<21.0	21.0–24.4	24.5–28.9	29.0–32.8	32.9–36.9	>36.9
50–59	<20.2	20.2–22.7	22.8–26.9	27.0–31.4	31.5–35.7	>35.7
60+	<17.5	17.5–20.1	20.2–24.4	24.5–30.2	30.3–31.4	>31.4

Male VO2 Max Levels

Age	Very Poor	Poor	Fair	Good	Excellent	Superior
13–19	<35.0	35.0–38.3	38.4–45.1	45.2–50.9	51.0–55.9	>55.9
20–29	<33.0	33.0–36.4	36.5–42.4	42.5–46.4	46.5–52.4	>52.4
30–39	<31.5	31.5–35.4	35.5–40.9	41.0–44.9	45.0–49.4	>49.4
40–49	<30.2	30.2–33.5	33.6–38.9	39.0–43.7	43.8–48.0	>48.0
50–59	<26.1	26.1–30.9	31.0–35.7	35.8–40.9	41.0–45.3	>45.3
60+	<20.5	20.5–26.0	26.1–32.2	32.3–36.4	36.5–44.2	>44.2

Table Reference: *The Physical Fitness Specialist Certification Manual*, The Cooper Institute for Aerobics Research, Dallas TX, revised 1997; printed in *Advance Fitness Assessment & Exercise Prescription*, 3rd Edition, Vivian H. Heyward, 1998, p.48.

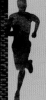

BLOCK 1
SLEEP

For most of my adult life I neither understood nor invested in the critical role of quality sleep and how to achieve it. But sleep is fundamental to mental and physical health and quality of life. Satisfying your body's sleep requirements is directly correlated to all aspects of mental and physical performance and aging. Sleep supports healthy brain function, growth and development, and it affects how well we think, react, work, learn and get along with others.

PROTECTING HEALTH

Sleep is the period when your body rests and repairs itself from the toils of your day. While every individual's sleep requirements are unique, we know most adults operate best within a 7–8-hour bracket. Physical exertion increases sleep requirements, in order for your body to adapt itself for subsequent sessions by repairing damaged tissue and increasing muscle fibres. Unfortunately, this is easier said than done, with the cumulative demands of modern family and professional life increasingly encroaching on this vital human need. Regardless, the costs associated with depriving our bodies from the sleep we need are severe. Even one poor night's sleep reduces immune system effectiveness, and prolonged sleep deficiency significantly increases the likelihood of a number of diseases. Sleep is also critical to your body's recovery and adaptation from training. Sleep supports training by increasing anabolic (muscle-building) hormones and decreasing catabolic (muscle-wasting) hormones.

AVERTING STRESS

Human evolutionary development is struggling to keep up with the world we now live in. Our bodies are unable to distinguish between physical and mental threats; both spur a fight-or-flight response. But whereas a physical threat channels energy towards activity – e.g. we either run from or kill the wild animal that invades our cave – emotional snipes that accompany office politics have no parallel or speedy resolution. The anxiety that accompanies these can be corrosive to sleep quality, which adds to the original stress. A dose of physical exertion is my trusted antidote to minor stresses – creating the conditions to metaphorically slay the wild animal.

AUGMENTING DECISION-MAKING

Sleep profoundly impacts behaviour and mental performance. During sleep the brain rids itself of waste products and creates synapses, by replaying and learning from the mental activity of the day. As with the muscle growth that occurs during sleep after physical exercise, the same is true of our brain: sleep both repairs the damage of the day and enhances its ability to solve the similar cognitive or emotional challenges for when they arise again. Optimal brain function is dependent on sufficient sleep: 7–8 hours. Deficiency inhibits our ability to think clearly, similar to being drunk,[*] and increases impulsive and risky behaviour. Poor sleep is correlated both to an increased tendency to gamble in decision-making and to take larger risks more frequently. Sleep deficit is linked to hedonic behaviour – prioritizing short-term fun and pleasure in decision-making often at the expense of long-term goals. A deficit of only 2 hours' sleep in one night results in effort discounting, meaning you avoid those things even remotely challenging. The cumulative effect of a deficit of 1–2 hours over a few days results in cognitive function impairment equal to a whole night missed. I am unable to think of any aspect of life in which heightened emotional reactivity and reduced cognitive control are positive traits. Indeed, any goal-focused

---

[*] As just one example, sleep deficiency while driving is attributed as the primary cause of more than 100,000 accidents per year and 1,500 road deaths in the US.

person – athlete, parent, business professional or all three – simply can't afford the performance cost and fallow time that follows. A total of 7–8 hours is the benchmark you need to aim for, adapting your training if this is not possible.

VIGILANCE AND NUTRITION

Sleep and nutrition are mutually supportive, but unfortunately deficiencies in one will also cannibalize the other. When we deprive our bodies of even a small amount of sleep, it increases the production of ghrelin, a hormone that makes us feel hungry, and reduces Leptin production, a hormone that makes us feel full. These biological chemical imbalances are further amplified by the effect sleep deprivation has on our decision-making as outlined above: a predisposition for hedonic behaviour, e.g. eating junk food, and an overactive reward centre, which reinforces the behaviour loop.

It's a diluted version of the behaviour that accompanies an ugly hangover. You desire high-fat, high-sugar food and drinks and the immediate feedback you receive from your body rewards you for doing so. Self-loathing may follow the behaviour pattern, but it doesn't happen soon enough to interrupt your decision-making. To be clear, it's not a lack of character, but a chemical imbalance caused by poor sleep that attacks the willpower to eat the right foods. In other words, making poor nutritional decisions is merely a symptom of sleep deficiency.

CIRCADIAN RHYTHM

The circadian rhythm describes a 24-hour cyclic activity. This synchronization ensures the right behaviour at the right time of day. We are efficient machines and have evolved to use only the parts of our body relevant for day or night activity, with more than 15% of our bodily functions regulated by our circadian rhythm. Unfortunately, with that efficiency comes challenge due to modern life. Less than 200 years ago, 90% of the global population worked outside in farming, with activity and sleep regulated by the season and daylight. Today 90% of the world's population live and work in light-regulated environments, where artificial light sends false messages to our body about the time of day. The single biggest assault on our circadian rhythms are our phones, which all too often accompany us to bed. The solution is self-evident but difficult to put into practice: we need to separate ourselves from the technologies that trick our bodies into thinking they should be awake when they need to be rejuvenating instead. Sleep like a caveman. Only your body knows how much sleep it needs; we help it by creating the conditions for our bodies to wake us after adequate rest, not in response to an alarm or light pollution. Optimizing our sleep starts with an early night and absence of technology at the bedside. Thereafter we need to kick start and anchor our circadian rhythm with sunlight, ideally starting the day with 30 minutes of outdoor exercise.

In summary, adequate sleep is fundamental to a productive life and an essential component of any health and fitness regime worthy of pursuit. **To be paratrooper fit, shoot for a 'straight 8' and *never* train on less than 7 hours' sleep**!

BLOCK 2
NUTRITION

The amount of information available on nutrition is confusing and frequently conflicting. What follows is not designed to be a comprehensive guide but a philosophy that seeks to dispel some myths and codify some principles for nutrition that will both support your training goals and be sustainable for the long term.

The Paratrooper Pyramid purposefully signposts that the return for an investment in nutrition offers far more than training alone. When faced with the choice of a well-constructed nutrition plan or a training plan of equal quality – pick nutrition first every time. Fortunately, this is not an either-or model; getting nutrition right first will maximize training results.

All my programmes will help you tone your body, lose fat and feel focused and energetic all day. In this section, however, my primary purpose is to outline a working approach and explain the connection between nutrition, fitness and health.

NUTRITION PLANNING

Remember: Nutrition accounts for 25% of performance. Meal planning/cooking time is disproportionate to the enjoyment derived from the activity. Reliance on convenience food will subvert nutrition and training goals.

How to start:
- Assign 3 hours for nutrition planning.
- Pick meals for 4-week rotation that support training goals/nutritional requirements, aiming for at least 5 breakfasts, 10 lunches, 15 dinners, 10 healthy snacks, 5 pre/post-training snacks; factor in hydration.
- Use 15 Nutritional Building Blocks to plan – see pages 51–54.
- Review ingredients with food types lists on page 49.
- Cross-reference with Fitness Standards table – see pages 145–146.
- Codify each week's shopping list and save online, to aid weekly food order.
- Codify perishable requirements to collect between online orders.
- Prepare in bulk, where possible – to reduce time spent preparing/cooking.
- Trial, review and optimize.

When you settle on a training programme in the later sections, it is essential that you **create a nutrition plan that fuels your body for success**, based on both your activity levels and your tastes. Only you can own the execution and the results.

Optimal Food Source
Green Vegetables: Asparagus • Garlic • Avocado • Onions • Beans • Kale • Broccoli • Mushrooms • Cabbage • Lettuce • Cauliflower • Olives • Celery • Spinach • Aubergine • Sugar Snap Peas • Green Peppers • Courgette
Proteins: Eggs • Fish & Seafood • Red Meat • Poultry – Chicken / Turkey
Fats: Butter • Olive Oil • Walnut Oil • Almond/Peanut Butter • Coconut Oil • Flaxseed Oil • Tahini • Ghee
Drinks: Water • Green & Herbal Tea • Black Tea • Lemon-Flavoured Water • Black Coffee
Sauces: Lemon & Lime Juice • Vinegar • Tamari • Mayonnaise (no added sugar) • Mustard • Tabasco or other chilli/pepper sauces
Herbs & Spices: Garlic • Basil • Cinnamon • Coriander • Ginger • Chilli • Cumin • Oregano • Sea Salt • Pepper • Paprika • Nutmeg • Turmeric
Seeds: Chia Seeds • Flax Seeds • Sunflower Seeds • Pumpkin Seeds

Foods to Consume More Selectively
Nuts: Limited to 30g a day. Almonds • Hazelnuts • Pine Nuts • Macadamia • Cashews • Walnuts • Nut Butters • Pistachios • Nut Milks • Peanuts
Whole Grains: Oats • Pumpernickel, Rye or Sourdough Bread • Wholemeal Pasta Red/Brown Rice • Quinoa Soba Noodles
Dairy: All Cheeses • Unsweetened Full-Fat Yoghurt
Pulses: Beans • Lupins • Lentils • Chickpeas
Starchy Vegetables: Corn • Potatoes • Pumpkins • Beetroot
Berries: Blueberries • Raspberries • Strawberries • Blackberries
Fruits: Apples • Oranges • Pears • Papayas • Melons • Kiwis
High Sugar Fruits: Bananas • Dried Fruits • Pineapples • Grapes
Foods to Avoid:
Refined Carbohydrates: Breakfast Cereals • White Noodles • White Pasta • White Wraps • Granola • White Flour • White Bread • White Rice
Sweets: Ice Cream • Sweets • Milk Chocolate • Cakes
Heart Killers: Heavily Processed Foods • Deep-Fried Foods

WATER

Water is vital for survival, let alone training. We need 3–4 litres a day to sustain moderate activity; drink less and we increase the risks of heat stroke, kidney disease, urinary tract infections, dry-eye disease, cataract formation, bladder and colon cancer, decreased immune function and constipation. We often confuse thirst with hunger, and as a result maintaining hydration has the added benefit of helping us avoid snacking unnecessarily. **Physical performance is significantly impaired by as little as 2% dehydration.** As we train hard, particularly in warmer climates, it is critical that we increase our water intake accordingly.

ANIMAL INSTINCTS

The point made earlier about the discord between our DNA and sleep holds true for the modern diet too. We evolved to sit at the top of the food chain through innovation and survival necessity, but it took us some time to get there and our metabolisms have yet to catch up. When we sat somewhere in the middle of that food chain, we ate leftovers of prey captured by other predators. We were foragers, eating wild animals and wild plants. Our diet was diverse and seasonal; so too were the times when we ate, often going days between meals. Today our diet

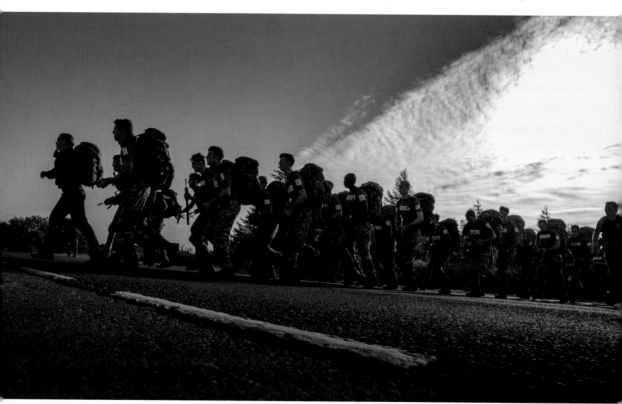

includes a plethora of staple foods that weren't in existence one generation ago, let alone 100,000 years ago. We'll hammer this point again: **processed carbohydrates and sugars are guilty pleasures** that should be treated like a recreational drug and rationed accordingly.

CALORIE COUNTING

Not all calories are created equal, and a simplistic focus on the energy content of food is not sufficient. Whether regulating your body weight to its optimal state or fuelling your body for performance in a specific domain, you must look beyond the calories. What's more important is how the calorie source affects our bodies' processing of the energy in the calorie; more specifically, the hormonal regulation of fat tissue. Much of what was previously advised by government health organizations was based on a false assumption that heart disease was caused by a diet high in saturated fats. This thinking led to the wholesale adoption of a diet high in carbohydrates and eradicating fats from our diet. An overwhelming body of research has since identified that when it comes to body fat regulation, carbohydrate calories, not fat, is what must be measured and controlled. Carbohydrates cause insulin secretion, which results in your body storing those calories as body fat. Restrict carbohydrates and your body mobilizes energy from fat reserves, a process referred to as ketosis. Furthermore, more energy is burned metabolizing calories from protein and fats; in addition, the body feels fuller after eating these food groups. The combined effect of a diet high in protein, fats and dietary fibre and low in carbohydrates is that insulin production is controlled, appetite is satisfied and more energy is expended during metabolism. As a general rule, when counting the macro nutrients of your diet, 20g per day of carbohydrates (high-quality) is optimal for regulating body fat, whereas 100g per day supports an active training programme for prospective paratroopers or amateur athletes. The timing of these meals is equally important, but we'll get to that later.

15 ESSENTIAL NUTRITIONAL BUILDING BLOCKS

1. **The mission determines resource allocation:** The demands placed on your body should be resourced sufficiently by your nutrition plan both in calorie and macro-nutrient terms. Wearable technology (smartphone/watch) makes it easy to determine your calorie consumption to within 10% accuracy. Our lives follow a rhythm, whether the repetitive cycle is the unit of a day, week or month. We know what constitutes normal activity and calorie expenditure, and our nutrition plan should be designed to support this, whether we're the one wearing

the oven gloves or otherwise. If eating out or business travel is standard, then we need an approach that proactively manages our consumption relative to any associated change in activity. All restaurants have menus – plan ahead. All airlines offer baggage allowances – take food with you.

2. **Log your nutrition:** You get what you measure; by recording your diet you can iterate and improve along the way. The evolution and ease of use of technology solutions such as myfitnesspal make capturing the macro ingredients of the foods alongside your activity easy, thereby ensuring you satisfying your body's requirements. Do this for a month and you'll quickly achieve a state where you're comfortable with what you get from specific meals and snacks; measurement and healthy decision-making will be intuitive.

3. **Abs are made in the shopping trolley:** The best way to avoid unhealthy food options is for them not to reside in your home. The solution is two-fold: purge them from your kitchen and banish them from your shopping trolley.

4. **Breakfast is king:** Breakfast is an essential component of your fuel plan. It kicks-starts the body and day for performance. If you train first thing, it may not be the first meal of the day, but it should never be skipped.

5. **Graze:** Grazing describes a practice of eating small meals throughout the day, which not only maintains energy levels but offsets the temptation of indulging on junk foods or quick fixes.

6. **Protein:** Muscle proteins are the building block for every muscle cell, and are made by the body from essential amino acids consumed in food. Each muscle cell undergoes a cycle of constant regeneration, fuelled by protein. The average sedentary person requires 0.8g of protein to support optimal body functioning, whereas active people require much more. To maximize the effectiveness of training, aim for 1–1.2g of protein per kg of bodyweight. An added benefit of protein is that it leaves you more satisfied than high-carb foods as well as boosting your metabolism. As an example, 100g of lean chicken breast contains 30g of protein. I use plant-based protein powder drinks as a great source of additional protein.

7. **Whole foods over processed:** Not all calories are created equal. You should always choose something that was once living (plant or animal) over a processed food whose origin is neither clear nor recent.

8. **Healthy snacks:** Often, it's the unplanned snack, not the pre-planned meals, which let us down with our nutrition. Create a selection of mobile

snacks that you can rotate throughout your plan to fend off hunger. Avocado, pine nuts, sunflower seeds, cashew nuts, almonds and full-fat Greek yoghurt are all great healthy choices.

9. **Fast daily:** The timing of when you eat and don't eat is important. Equally, ensuring you eat within an 11–13 hour window promotes ketosis, your body's ability to readily access its body fat storage as an energy source. Monday to Friday I frequently confine my eating to an 8-hour window and feel great for doing so.

10. **Fruit and vegetables:** Both fruits and vegetables are great sources of fibre, antioxidants and phytonutrients. Notwithstanding the botanical differences, the main distinction is that fruit has a much higher sugar content, with grapes, bananas and dates topping the natural sugar charts. Green vegetables have the least sugar content. Sugar, even that found in fruit, must be rationed sensibly to avoid it cannibalizing your health and training goals – less is more. Fruit juices are particularly noxious and should generally be avoided as they contain all of the fruit sugar and none of the fibre that would normally help your body metabolize it.

11. **Restrict alcohol:** Like sugar, alcohol consumption should be controlled closely. The benefits of a glass of red wine on longevity are well telegraphed, and the resveratrol contained within it is a recognized cancer killer. Notwithstanding this, most alcoholic drinks, especially beer, are full of sugar and empty calories.

12. **Omega 3:** There are many health benefits associated with eating foods rich in omega 3 fatty acids, such as reducing the incidence of heart disease, anxiety, inflammation and metabolic syndrome, to name but a few. It's available naturally in eggs and fish, but other foods such as butters are now having them added to enhance them. Two portions of fish per week is your best source and should be included in your diet.

13. **Fuel exercise:** Optimum performance and optimum recovery are fuelled by food and water. In order to maximize the benefits from training, it's important to consciously fuel your session, ensuring it's aligned to your training goals.

    a. **Water:** The best way to determine the water requirements of an hour's training activity is to weigh yourself naked before and after the session. The differential in kg is the water you lost while training that needs replenishing. Multiply this by the number of hours spent training for the total bill. For activities in warmer climates this may exceed your body's ability to process the water

(1.2–1.5 litres per hour), in which case you will need to add salt tablets so it can be adsorbed.

b. **Strength training:** Powerlifters and bodybuilders are adept at calibrating their protein consumption to maximize its effectiveness. To propel your strength training to the next level, incorporate 20–40g of protein 20 minutes before and after your session, with 5g of BCAA amino acids[*] to support muscle recovery and growth.

c. **Cardiovascular training:** Depending on the intensity of your session, 1–2 hours can be fuelled by the body's glycogen stores, which contain 2,000 calories of readily available energy. An active endurance runner needs approximately 1–1.3g of carbohydrates per kg of bodyweight. As an example, 100g of sweet potato contains 20g of carbohydrates.

14. **Minimize sugar:** Our bodies crave and enjoy sugar, and it is the single biggest source of weight gain thanks to its addictive qualities. Whether lurking in a soft drink, sweet breakfast cereal or seemingly healthy piece of fruit, it creates a spike in your insulin level that triggers a slowdown in your metabolism and ultimately results in your body storing the calories as fat.

15. **Consistency:** The best nutrition plan is irrelevant without consistent application. Blow-outs will happen, but most can be anticipated and either avoided or embraced as a well-deserved break. It's easier to apply something 100% of the time than 99% of the time, but there will always be mission creep in your exception criteria – I always (and only) eat cake at birthdays!

BLOCK 3
MOBILITY

The human body is a complex machine, which if correctly organized and fully functioning should act in harmony. Mobility is moving safely to maximize physical potential. It has two building blocks: motor control and range of motion. Motor control is the technique, conscious or otherwise, for moving your body as it was designed to do. Range of motion is the freedom of movement available in a joint.

---

[*] Three essential amino acids that must be obtained from food, as your body cannot produce them.

SUPRESS INJURY

Unfortunately, the real symptoms of poor mobility appear all too late, which often means the first time you're aware of a problem is when something breaks. To make matters worse, pain is less noticeable during high stress and peak exertion. In other words, our bodies' fight or flight response hasn't evolved quickly enough to tell the difference between running from a predator or in a training session; for both it shuts out all other signals to focus on the task at hand, so injuries go unnoticed. Add a well-intended 'no pain, no gain' attitude and it is a recipe for disaster. I would liken poor mobility to driving a car with a flat tyre; you may get away with it a few times, but it will quickly become expensive. Our bodies were designed for millions of movement cycles, but just like the flat tyre, every movement done sub-optimally burns through those cycles quicker. This issue doesn't just apply to the gym; even the most sedentary existence, if executed with poor posture, cannibalizes your body's useful lifespan. Put simply, your body will eventually refuse to slouch in a chair and lift with a rounded back and it's unlikely it will give you a second chance with either.

TRAIN FOR LIFE

The combination of advances in training and access to information made possible by technological advances has promoted a consciousness of mobility even at amateur-level sport which a decade ago would have been restricted to those competing in the world gymnastics arena. Our aim from training is not to identify an exhaustive list of mobility issues to fix, but rather use training as a means of perfecting motor control, range of motion and efficiency. All of the training programmes in this book provide a vocabulary of movements that will flag any mobility deficiencies you have at the same time as progressively enhancing your base level of mobility.

I have designed the PARA Fit training programmes to optimize mobility by focusing on seven basic primal movement patterns: **squat**, **lunge**, **push**, **pull**, **twist**, **bend** and **gait** (walk, run, crawl),* activities that prioritize spinal mechanics and full ranges of motion. In essence, the training programmes will work to strengthen and develop your mobility, thus helping avoid injury, not only in the gym but at home and in your workplace.

---

* Chek, P. *How to Eat, Move and Be Healthy! Your Personalized 4-Step Guide to Looking and Feeling Great from the Inside Out.* C.H.E.K Institute, 2004.

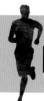

FUNCTION ASSESSMENT

The following seven functional movement screen assessments should be undertaken before starting your fitness journey. Lower functional movement scores significantly increase your risk of injury. I strongly recommend you start and remain on the first programme (Boot Camp – see pages 106–109) until you have achieved level 2 in at least five of the seven assessments. Subject to your current mobility point, the Boot Camp programme will get you level 2 in all seven tests in a few four-week cycles if followed diligently.

OVERHEAD SQUAT

Level 1

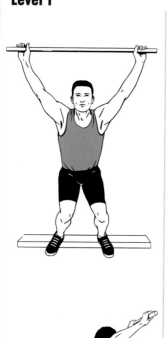

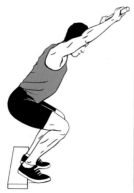

Level 2

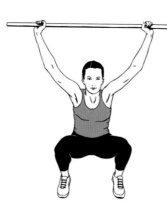

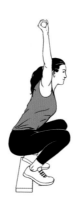

Level 3

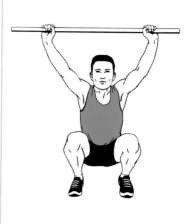

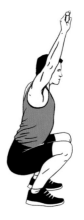

INLINE LUNGE
Level 1   **Level 2**   **Level 3**

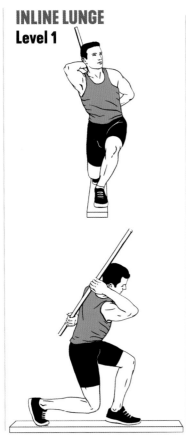

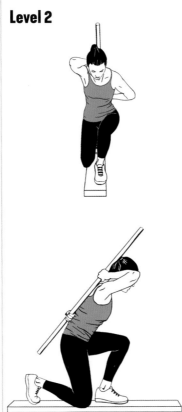

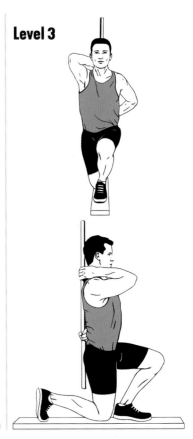

SHOULDER MOBILITY
Level 1   **Level 2**   **Level 3**

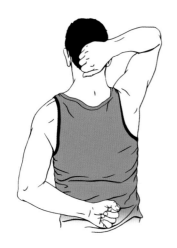

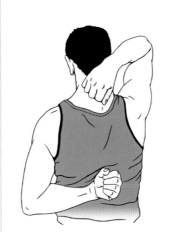

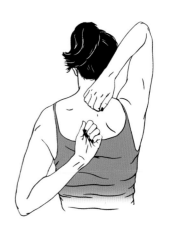

HURDLE STEP
Level 1   Level 2   Level 3

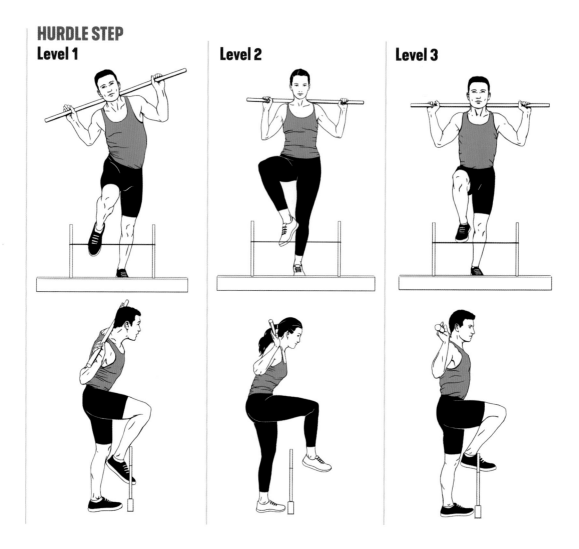

ACTIVE STRAIGHT LEG RAISE
Level 1   Level 2

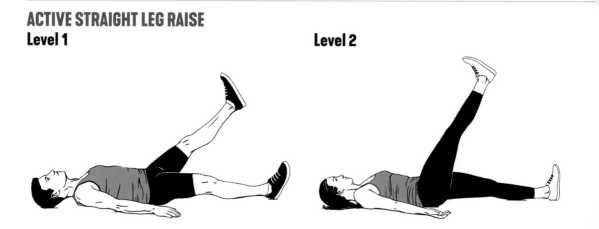

ROTARY STABILITY
Level 1

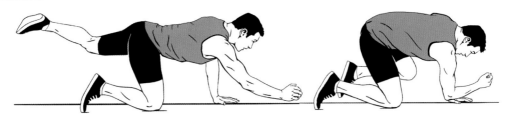

Level 2

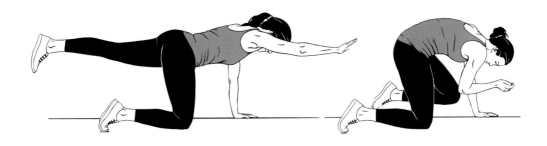

Level 3

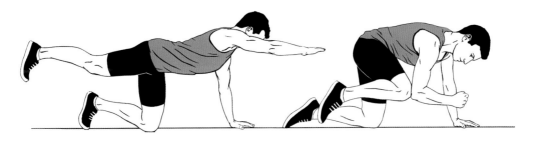

Level 3

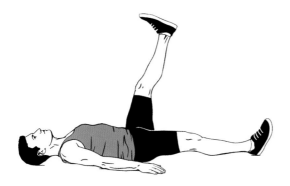

TRUNK STABILITY PUSH-UP
Level 1

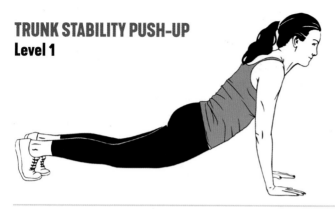

Level 2

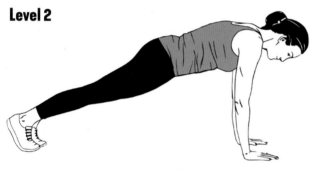

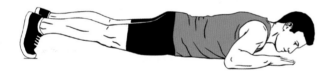

Level 3

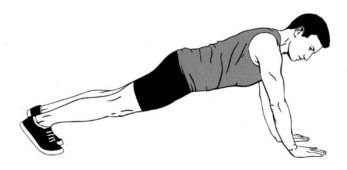

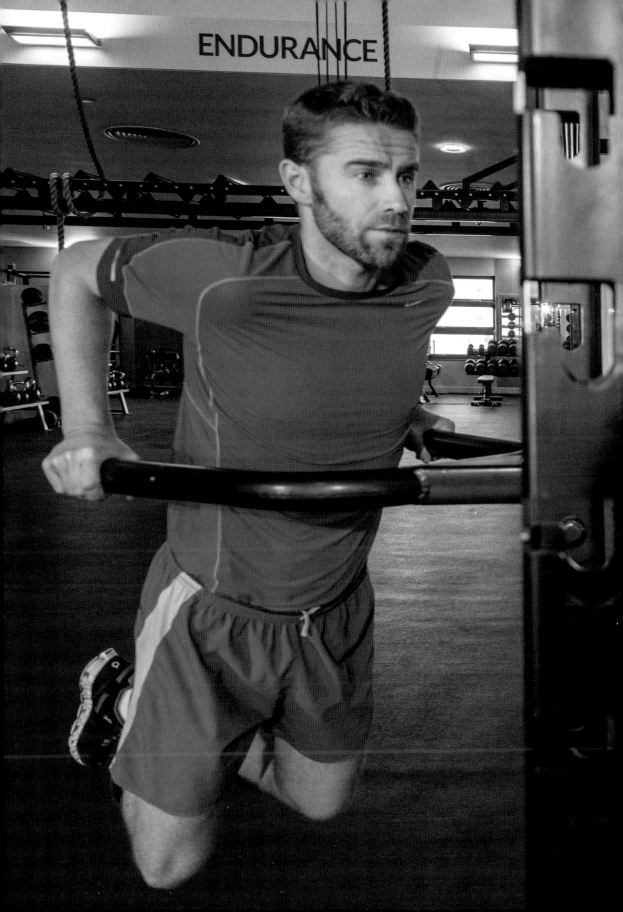

ESSENTIALS OF THE PARA FIT APPROACH

TRAINING VS EXERCISE

Training is an approach focused on aligning each component of the system to achieve optimal performance, whereas exercise is an activity done for its own sake. Paratroopers train to be the best possible expression of themselves – so should you.

THE PARATROOPER PYRAMID: SYSTEMIZED TRAINING

The paratrooper training approach is about focusing effort. A programme that emphasizes the gym and neglects sleep, nutrition and mobility is the fast track to mediocrity and ultimately demotivation. Sleep, nutrition and mobility offer significantly more leverage than any amount of purposeful training you will do. The higher you set your training goals, the more compromises to sleep, nutrition and mobility will corrode your progress.

1. **Sleep.** Fundamental to functioning both mentally and physically. Sleep fuels recovery. Aim for 8 hours, but never train on less than 7 hours of sleep.
2. **Nutrition.** The optimum nutrition plan is high in water and whole foods and as plant based as possible, with alcohol and sugar treated like guilty pleasures. It is impossible to train your way out of a bad diet and nothing will cannibalize your goals quicker.
3. **Mobility.** Optimal mobility enables your body to act in harmony and maximizes physical potential. Training while neglecting mobility is the quickest route to injury.

All pyramids require a strong base. To explore the summit of your pyramid, sleep, hydration, mobility and nutrition are more important than anything you'll do in the gym. The next section will be focused on the tactics necessary to reach the summit, but it will be irrelevant if you ignore the base.

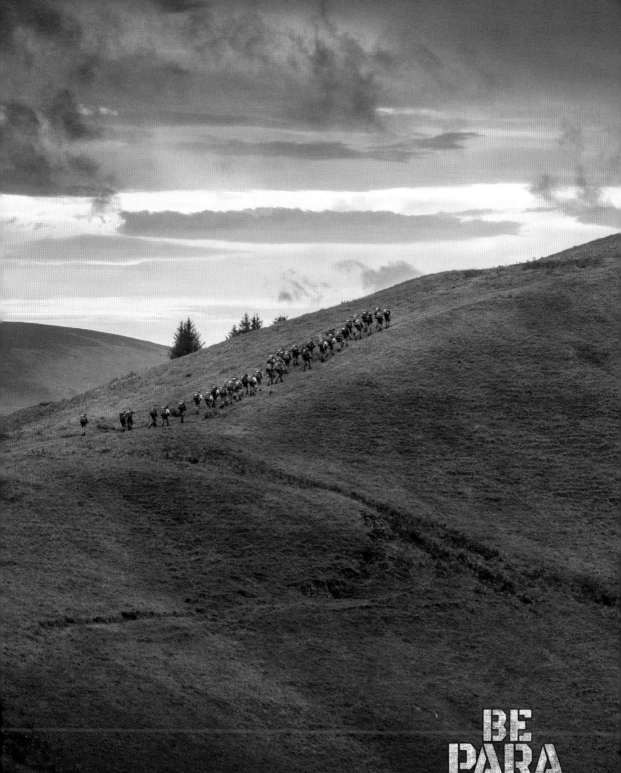

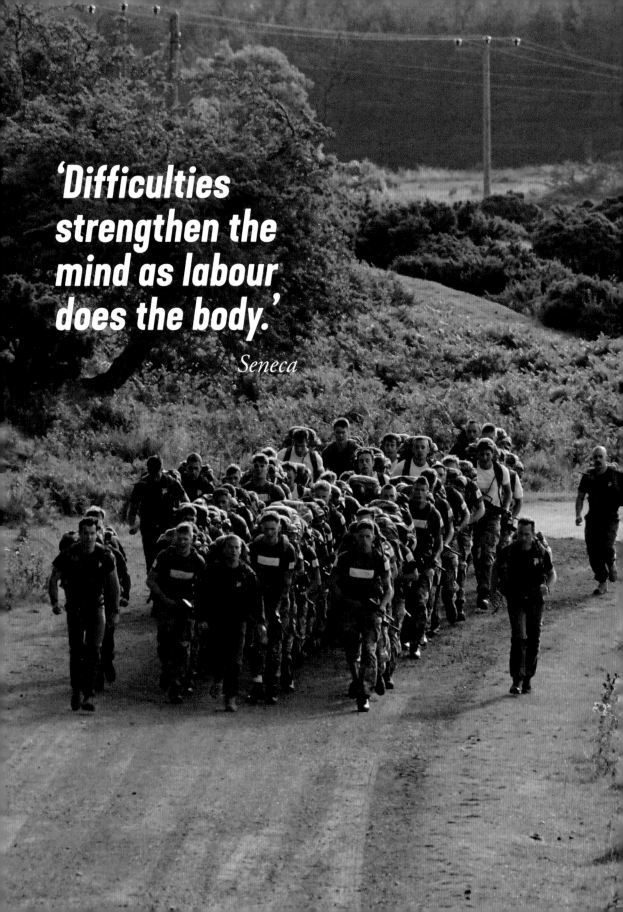

'Difficulties strengthen the mind as labour does the body.'

Seneca

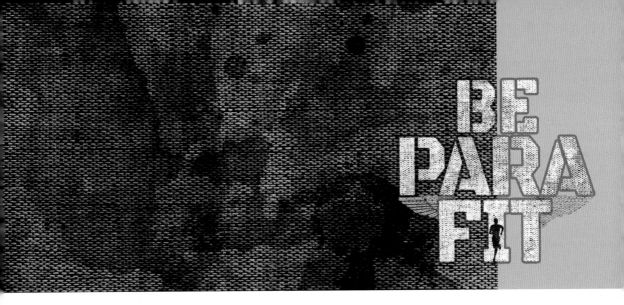

CHAPTER 3

PARA FIT TRAINING PRINCIPLES

In this chapter, my intention is not only to equip you with a training programme but also with the theory underpinning it. To achieve your physical potential you will need to master the training process, so you can eventually build your own programmes tailored to your chosen stretch goal. But far more important in the short term is understanding why the regime you're embarking on will succeed.

COMPONENTS OF FITNESS

An effective training programme is organized to efficiently address the specific needs of the individual, to help them bridge the gap between their current state and desired physical state. In the *Be PARA Fit* training programmes we will use a fitness assessment at the start of every four-week training cycle, to assess first your starting point and then your progress along the way. Advancement is competency-based; to progress you must master each incremental step. The building blocks of all physical training are strength, speed and agility, and endurance.

STRENGTH

Strength is an essential physical attribute, which positively affects all other components of fitness. Greater strength supports skill development, complex movements (e.g. jumping, sprinting, changing direction), robustness and resilience and reduces risk of injury. Strength can be further broken down into:

- maximal strength – the maximum force a muscle can exert in a single contraction;
- explosive strength – the acceleration of force a muscle can exert;
- muscular endurance – the ability of a muscle to sustain repeated contractions against some form of resistance for an extended period of time.

In the PARA Fit programmes we use functional movements with either weights or body weight to improve strength.

SPEED AND AGILITY

Speed is the ability to cover a distance quickly. Speed is multidimensional, since it relates to and supports the development of a multitude of other physical abilities.

Agility is the ability to coordinate movement skills with speed, balance, spatial awareness and decision-making. Agility improves mobility, flexibility and coordination.

In the PARA Fit programmes speed and agility are honed through acceleration, deceleration and turning when running and in the functional movements such as jumping, burpees and deadlifts.

ENDURANCE

Endurance is the ability to maintain or to repeat a given force or power output. It has two components which relate to the energy systems that fuel the activity: aerobic (with oxygen) and anaerobic (without oxygen).

In the PARA Fit programmes endurance is developed using longer training sessions, such as distance running/cycling, etc. Shorter sessions such as tempo training, interval training and circuit training also all improve endurance.

TRAINING ADAPTATION

Performance in training is achieved through a cycle of **stress**, **recovery** and **adaptation**. Stress is characterized by a trigger that causes a physiological change, disrupting the body's normal state. Recovery is the body's way of preserving itself by returning to its pre-stress state, enhanced for when the stress reoccurs. Adaptation is the body's way of enduring an evolving environment. Training seeks to optimize this cycle, by tailoring stress and recovery to your physical capabilities so you achieve your potential as quickly as possible.

Progress is quick and easy for the novice, slow and complex for the expert. For the complete beginner every session exerts a stress sufficient to create adaptation by the next workout. The markings of the end of a novice phase are a performance plateau, requiring more focused activities to maintain a positive performance trajectory. Unplanned exercise activities may get you this far, but no further. Elite athletic performance not only involves enormous physical and social costs, but it also requires the complex manipulation of training and other parameters, tailored to the individual athlete.

FOUR BUILDING BLOCKS OF TRAINING

Whatever your fitness goal, there are four basic principles that are the building blocks of every training programme, and which ultimately will determine how quickly and successfully you will achieve your training targets. These are:

1. **Frequency** – how often you train. While generally the more you train the quicker you will improve, it is possible to over-train, which can limit your progress.
2. **Intensity** – how hard you train. The aim is to progressively push your body using incremental steps.
3. **Time** – how long you train for. This should be based on the type of activity you are engaged in and your training goal. For people returning to exercise or working towards a new goal, the time spent exercising should be increased as personal fitness develops.
4. **Type** – the type of exercise undertaken. According to training principles, the type of exercise conducted is derived from the aim of the training session or programme.

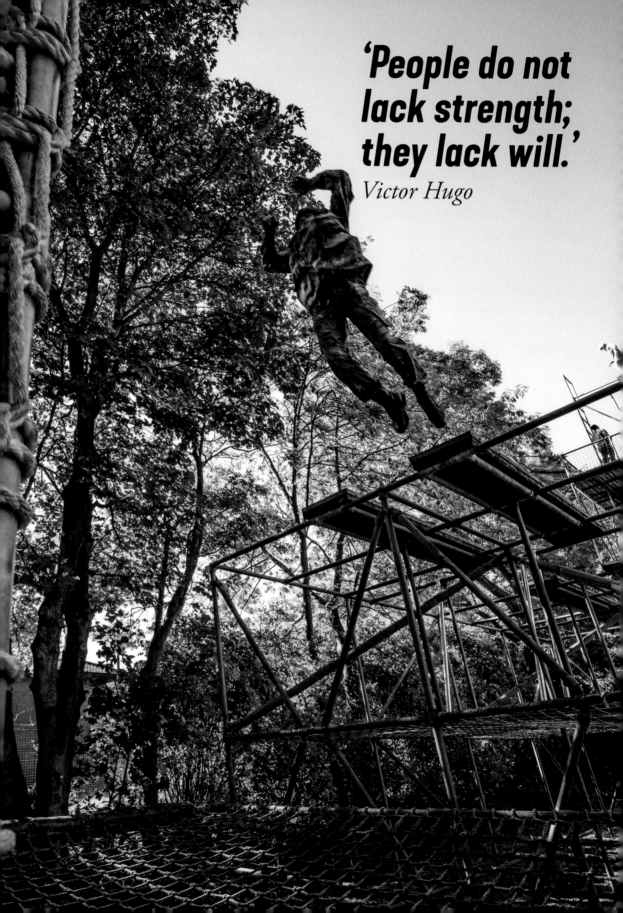

'People do not lack strength; they lack will.'
Victor Hugo

OVER-TRAINING AND EFFECTIVE RECOVERY

While overloading the body is the very process by which the body adapts and gets fitter, without adequate recovery it becomes self-defeating. Exhaustion is the cumulative effect of over-training and occurs when the frequency, intensity and time spent training causes sufficient stress to exceed the body's ability to adapt adequately.

Rest, and specifically sleep, are key allies. As detailed in Chapter 2, 7–8 hours' sleep is essential to support training development. Recovery becomes particularly important during intense training or competition periods to sustain an optimal state of performance. Recovery is multi-dimensional, with multiple other factors impacting your body's ability to rejuvenate, such as nutrition, stress, your health and your local environment. Understanding the importance of recovery has led to the use and development of many recovery techniques, including the following.

ACTIVE RECOVERY

Active recovery involves periods of low-intensity exercise performed between heavy training sessions or between competitions, to enhance the recovery process. A recovery run is a type of run normally done by endurance runners after a competition or during a period of intense training. It is important to ensure that recovery runs don't turn into junk miles. The aim of these runs is to flush out waste products, not add unnecessary miles to your training programme. Recovery runs (60% max heart rate) feature in the de-load weeks of the programmes.

Benefits:
- promotes blood flow and replenish glycogen stores in muscles;
- helps reduce build-up of waste products post-exercise;
- improves range of motion and motor control;
- aids in injury prevention.

Key points:
- normally used day after competition or particularly demanding session;
- mode is low-intensity, low-impact, cardiovascular exercise designed to assist in the recovery process;
- fitness development not priority of session;
- duration 30 minutes and below.

COLD WATER IMMERSION (ICE BATHS)

Cold-water therapy is a recovery process involving the immersion of the body into cold water immediately after exercise. While ice baths are not mandated within any of the PARA Fit programmes, I would recommend using them following races or competitions to help speed up recovery. Where possible I use an ice bath following a training run or race of more than 40km to aid my recovery.

Benefits:
- removes waste products from body;
- improves cardiovascular circulation;
- reduces muscle inflammation and damage;
- improves full range of movement.

Key points:
- optimal temperature is 11–12 degrees Celsius (52–54 degrees Fahrenheit);
- submersion of 1–2 minutes, repeated 3–4 times, with 30 seconds between submersions;
- improvised method of using ice cubes in a home bath is just as effective and requires approximately 10kg of ice.

COMPRESSION GARMENTS

Compression garments are tight, compressive forms of clothing, often made out of elastin and nylon, which are designed to enhance recovery. I typically sleep in compression tights following a big race and often wear compression calf sleeves.

Benefits:
- removes waste products in muscles;
- increases blood flow locally;
- reduces muscle movement during training.

COMMON INJURIES

SPRAINED ANKLE
- **Cause:** An over-stretching or tearing of supporting ligaments.
- **Symptoms:** Local inflammation, pain and bruising.
- **Prevention:** Careful footing over uneven terrain. Improve ligament strength using leg-balancing exercises. Try standing on one leg and throwing a ball against a wall using alternate hands.

ILIOTIBIAL BAND (ITB) SYNDROME
- **Cause:** Lazy gluteal muscles and poor pre- and post-exercise stretch discipline.
- **Symptoms:** Acute pain in the vicinity of the kneecap while running.
- **Prevention:** Comprehensive warm-up and cool down before and after exercise and glute strengthening exercises. If suffered, try rowing with a resistance band tied just above your knee.

ACHILLES TENDONITIS
- **Cause:** Over-training, badly fitting shoes and poor stretching regime.
- **Symptoms:** Inflammation and tenderness at the back of the heel.
- **Prevention:** Calf stretching before and after exercise, ensuring sufficient rest between sessions and wearing the right footwear. If sustained, spend as much time as you can stretching and massaging the area and avoid activities which aggravate the symptoms.

SHIN SPLINTS
- **Cause:** Over-training, following a programme with too much impact or not changing running shoes frequently enough.
- **Symptoms:** A dull ache felt along the front of the shin bone.
- **Prevention:** Alternating between high- and low-impact training sessions during your training programme and changing running shoes regularly. If developed, use alternative exercises until the symptoms disappear.

MUSCLE TEARS
- **Cause:** Over-training, hyperextension from a sudden movement, or too many repetitions of the same exercise.
- **Symptoms:** Feeling a sudden, painful tearing sensation which turns into an acute pain in the muscle.
- **Prevention:** Thorough warm-up and stretching before working out and taking care to gradually increase the frequency and intensity of sessions. If suffered, rest and engage in activities that exercise different parts of the body.

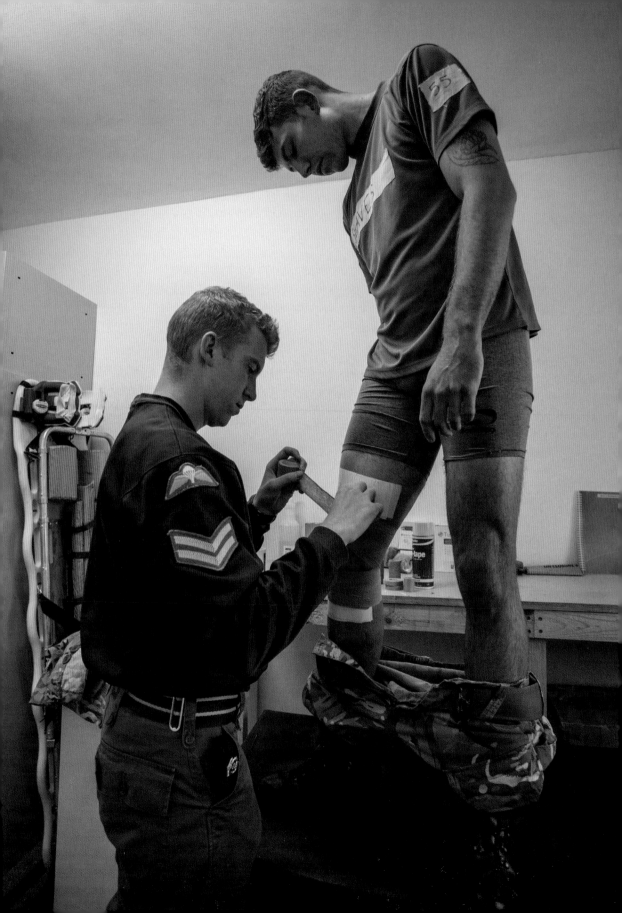

KIT AND EQUIPMENT

Some people say that a good workman never blames his tools, but find me a good workman who uses bad ones! Paratroopers pride themselves on looking after their kit, because on operations even the simplest items have the ability to transform, or even save, your life. The importance of maintaining kit is instilled in soldiers during Parachute Regiment training. The wrong, or badly fitting, kit makes even the most moderate of tasks impossible. Having experienced the effects of badly fitting boots and a poorly packed Bergen, these are not mistakes I will repeat. In a physical training environment the wrong kit can cause injuries that unhinge your entire training programme. The following list is by no means exhaustive, but it will give you an idea of what is important and what you can do without.

TRAINING SHOES

Your training shoes are perhaps the most important element of your fitness kit; therefore, it is worth investing time and money to make sure you get the right ones for you. As a general rule it is best to go to a specialist sports shop to be fitted for a shoe that meets all your requirements. However, if you're not able to do this, here are some tips.

- **Size matters:** Your feet swell during exercise, so consider getting shoes half a size larger than your normal ones. Also, take particular care in ensuring that the shoe is wide enough as well as long enough.
- **Cushioning:** When you run, your training shoe has to absorb three times your body weight. If you are a heavy runner, or have a history of compression injuries, find a training shoe with extra cushioning.
- **Fit for the task:** You need to select a training shoe which is appropriate for the surface you will mostly be running on. Whether you are road running, off-road running or a combination of the two, find a shoe which is designed for the purpose. If in doubt, find a hybrid trainer, which will have a tread deep enough to cope with running both on and off road.
- **Replacing your shoes:** As you would expect, the more you run, the more often you will need to change your shoes. As a rule you should aim to change your trainers every 500–600 miles.
- **How much?:** This depends entirely on your ego. While your knees will absorb the cost of a cheap pair of trainers, the most expensive pair won't necessarily be the best. I believe going to a specialist shop is worth the investment for your first pair; thereafter I'd suggest buying your next pair (of the same model) online.

CLOTHING

Good clothes won't turn a shire horse into a thoroughbred, but they will make you feel more comfortable and, therefore, more likely to train.

- **Shorts:** Whatever your preferred style, find shorts that are made of a lightweight and breathable material. Select a size and style that will reduce chafing between your legs. However, if you do suffer from this, Vaseline is another good solution.
- **Tops:** Like your shorts, you are looking for a top which is lightweight, breathable and made of a material that will wick the sweat away from your body. Once you have taken those criteria into

consideration, the style you choose is really a combination of personal preference and finding something appropriate for your training environment.

- **Leggings:** I think running leggings are brilliant. They are much lighter than tracksuit bottoms, but keep you just as warm.
- **Jackets:** Running in winter can be made much more bearable with the right jacket. Look for a breathable, waterproof jacket which will not only keep you dry, but also provide a barrier against the wind.
- **Socks:** While I am prone to going without socks, they do provide a barrier that protects your feet against rubbing and your shoes from stinking. It is possible to spend a lot on a pair of technical socks that offers anti-blister protection, extra cushioning or aids circulation, but I think it is better to find a pair that is comfortable and within your price range.

OTHER ITEMS

- **Watch:** You need a watch to keep track of how long you are training for. You don't need anything fancy and a good starting point is a waterproof watch with a stopwatch, lap counter and countdown facility. Until recently I ran with an Apple watch, which also acted as my heart rate monitor, music player and GPS. I have subsequently switched to a Garmin Fenix5X running watch, which I find is better placed to track my training and other health data.
- **Foam roller:** You need a foam roller to perform self-myofascial release (SMR)/foam rolling, which releases muscle tightness or trigger points. Once a mysterious technique exclusively used by professional athletes and therapists, with a small investment in a foam roller this everyday practice can transform muscle stiffness and your recovery from training. Foam rollers come in all shapes, sizes and budgets. Personally, I use a bamboo roller with a foam jacket.
- **Pull-up bar:** All but the Boot Camp programme use pull-ups – it is easily my favourite compound functional exercise. You will need a pull-up bar when you progress to these programmes. Pull-up bars are cheap (£10) and will fit on any door frame.
- **Kettle bell:** The PARA Fit programme uses single-leg Romanian deadlifts. As your strength develops you may want to include a weight instead of more repetitions to increase the intensity. I would recommend using a 12kg or 16kg kettle bell. Kettlebells are modestly priced (£20) and readily available online.
- **Music:** Definitely in the non-essential bucket, but music is great company on a hard workout. I love music and enjoy an equal mix of training with or without it. Whether on my Wattbike or during long, slow runs, I find a podcast or audio book helps keep things interesting when the scenery isn't, particularly if I'm doing a long stairs session. If running with a small running rucksack or belt, a phone with cord earphones works well, but my personal preference is wireless earphones connected to my watch.
- **Bergen (rucksack):** If your destination is the Parachute Regiment and you're using the P Company programme you'll need a military Bergen or at least a robust rucksack. The current British military-issue Bergen can be purchased online or from army surplus stores.

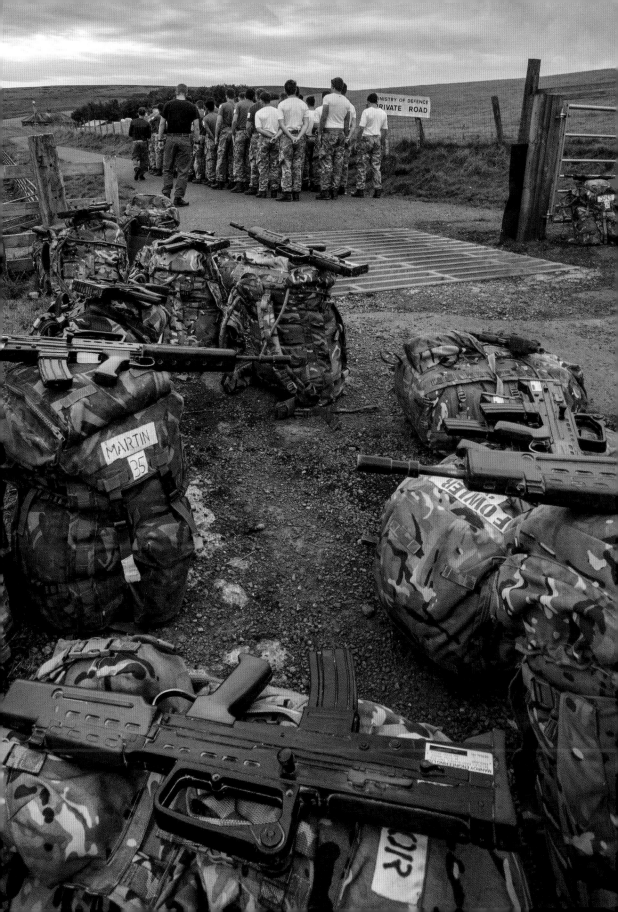

TRAINING PRINCIPLES IN BRIEF

INDIVIDUAL NEEDS
Training should be tailored to the individual's goal and starting point using the building blocks of strength, speed and agility, and endurance to create and constantly improve your training programme.

TRAINING ADAPTATION
Training works by inducing a cycle of stress, recovery and adaptation. Stress triggers physiological change, which takes place while sleeping and results in the body repairing damaged tissue so it is better prepared to perform the activity again. Subject to the fitness level of the athlete, this cycle takes 24–72 hours.

OVER-TRAINING
A tell-tale sign of over-training is the body not recovering from training within 72 hours. Listen to your body!

DIMINISHING RETURNS
Progress for the novice athlete is quick and fast, but as fitness improves each increment becomes slower and harder to realize so don't lose heart.

RECOVERY
Recovery is fundamental to every training cycle, during which the body adapts. There are multiple factors such as psychological stress, lifestyle, health and environment which impact recovery. There also are various techniques, such as active recovery and compression garments, that can be applied to enhance recovery.

The next section details the PARA Fit programmes, all of which have been designed using the training principles described above. To maintain progress and maximize training effectiveness, training programmes should seek to manipulate the stress, recovery, adaptation cycle. Four weeks represents the standard training cycle, with three stress (load) weeks, followed by one recovery (de-load) week.

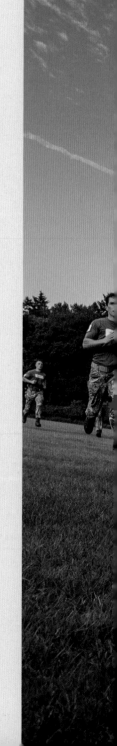

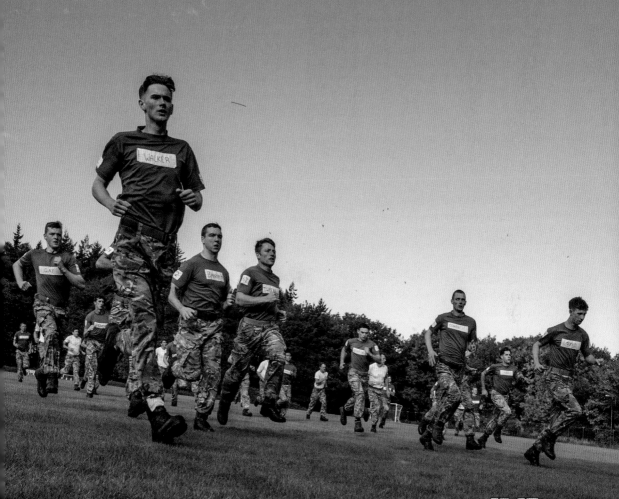

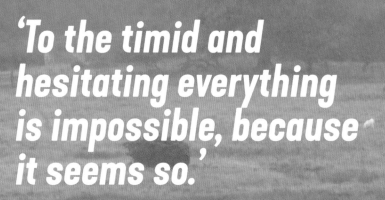

'To the timid and
hesitating everything
is impossible, because
it seems so.'

Sir Walter Scott

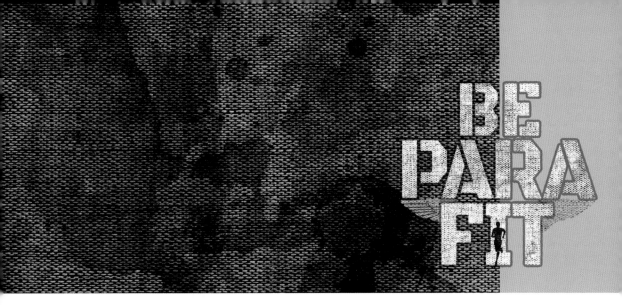

Chapter 4

TRAINING PROGRAMMES

Standard Operating Procedures (SOPs) are critical to the effective performance of paratroopers and other military personnel. Essentially, SOPs are a careful set of instructions on how to tackle just about any task a paratrooper might encounter. The master SOP of any PARA unit is its **battle rhythm**, which relates to both the format and tempo of all tasks, however big or small. Like a fighter's stance, the **battle rhythm provides the stability and balance to evolve, adapt and align to the inevitable challenges that arise in a dynamic and hostile environment.** A refined battle rhythm makes sustained and extended operations not only possible, but more likely to succeed because what has worked in the past has been refined; what has not has been discarded.

I have used the same key principle in my fitness programme design. Applying this principle to training is extremely potent; the more you make training routine, the better you're able to optimize *all* other activities to complement your training and remove friction.

TRAINING LEVELS AND THE FOUR-WEEK CYCLE

Each of the programmes detailed below has been tailored to develop your fitness, starting at the level you are at now. The programmes can be done individually to improve and maintain your desired level of fitness, but ultimately the aim is to make you 'PARA Fit', with the final programme intended specifically for those considering embarking on the Paratrooper Selection Course. Six hours is the maximum time needed to train per week. By repeating training patterns on a four-week rotation and doing the same type of activity every day of the week (e.g. Monday and Thursday are always strength days), **we will be able to build habits within just one four-week cycle**. While each programme has mobility built into the curriculum, as outlined in Chapter 2, we will quadruple training effectiveness by concurrently supporting your sleep and nutritional requirements. The programmes are arranged incrementally and categorized as follows:

- **Level 1 – Boot Camp:** Designed for those new to fitness or returning to it. This programme will systematically improve mobility alongside strength and aerobic fitness. Based on your starting point it may take multiple four-week cycles of this programme till you're ready to graduate to Level 2.
- **Level 2 – Fighting Fit:** For those already active, but at a rudimentary level. This programme will build on the foundations developed in Level 1. With disciplined focus, after a few patterns of this programme you should be at a standard to start the PARA Fit programme.
- **Level 3 – PARA Fit**: Don't be fooled by the simplicity of this programme. If followed precisely it will spur even those with a high base level of fitness to struggle and evolve on a continuous cycle of improvement. On entering this programme, I would expect it to take five to ten four-week cycles to get you to this Paratrooper standard of fitness, provided you make the right investments in sleep and nutrition.
- **P Company:** Designed primarily for those wishing to embark on Paratrooper selection for the British Parachute Regiment, but also for anyone who is aiming to add another dimension to their training regime. Its entry point is the same as PARA Fit, but it incorporates course-specific training, such as running in boots with a rucksack, to drive the grit necessary to thrive in P Company.

In the Boot Camp programme, all you will need is your training attire. In all other programmes you will need access to either a modest gym or a pull-up bar two days a week. For the P Company programme you will also require a rucksack and military-style boots.

There is a table of performance standards on page 83 to help you decide which starting point is best for you.

INTRODUCTION TO PARA FIT TRAINING

As highlighted above, each programme is a four-week cycle of progressive intensity. As you get fitter, the standards to achieve on week four determine whether you graduate to the next programme or increase the intensity for the next cycle of your current one. Here are the essential components:

Time frame. All training sessions are designed to be completed within an hour,* meaning that even at the highest level all you need is a maximum of six hours a week. The elegance of these four programmes lies in their comprehensiveness and simplicity – within three to five sessions you will have engrained the programme to memory and it will become an instinctive drill.

Mobility. We use the same mobility patterns for warm-ups, with a subset of these same exercises to cool down. At first you should aim to hold each position for as long as you can, striving for 30 seconds, which, once possible, becomes the standard for each session.

Circuit training. You can use the gym and non-gym based functional movements interchangeably. Getting your form right will be key. Regardless of how easy you find it, start with light weights for the first three sessions and work on your form – ideally get a trained eye to observe you and provide feedback. Add weight slowly and never train through a niggle.

Intensity gauge. The intensity for the strength sessions is 70%, the sweet spot for muscular growth. You will have got it right if you're able to complete the same number of reps (8–10) in the first two sets, but fall short by a few on your final set (e.g. 5–6).

Cardiovascular training. We deploy light cardio activity in the first level of the programme and progress to interval, threshold and fuel efficiency training in subsequent levels. Each of these sessions can be undertaken either by running, rowing or swimming subject to your preference. Intensity guidelines correspond to the Cardio Training Effort table on page 98.

---

* The exception is the P Company programme, which includes an up-to-2hr Bergen session to prepare those aspiring for Parachute Regiment selection for the P Company 10-miler.

Periodization: We leverage the principles of periodization, a long-term cyclic structuring of training, to maximize performance. We do this by controlling the degree of stress placed on the body, through the manipulation of the volume and intensity, in order to promote adaptation and development. As a result all programmes follow a cadence of three load weeks followed by one de-load week.

SELECTING YOUR STARTING POINT

If you're well versed in fitness, review the performance standards that follow and pick the programme that you think suits you best. Then take the fitness assessment on day 1 (see pages 56–60) and test and adjust based on how you get on. You may well be at different standards for different disciplines. We cater for this in the Be PARA Fit app, so your programme is tailored to your current level across all activities. If you're not currently using the Be PARA Fit app why not download it to help you customize your training to your personal fitness needs? Otherwise, proceed by picking the most relevant modules (cardio and circuit training) from each programme level that correspond to your standards – e.g. combining cardio sessions from the Be PARA Fit programme with circuit training sessions from the Fighting Fit programme.

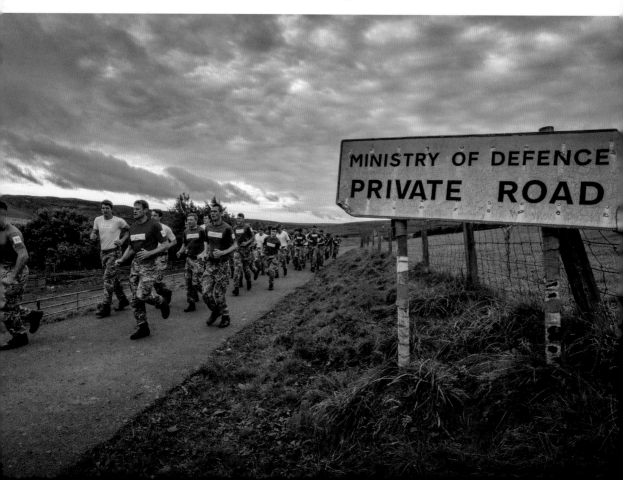

Male Performance Standards

Cardiovascular Fitness Activity (Pick 1 of 3)	Level 1	Level 2	Level 3	Paratrooper
Running / Rowing				
2.4km	>12.31 mins	10.30–12.30 mins	8.30–10.31 mins	Under 8.00 mins
10km	>55 mins	44–55 mins	38–43.59 mins	Under 38 mins
16km	>87 mins	75–87 mins	65–75 mins	Under 65 mins
Swimming				
750m	>20 mins	13.30–19.59 mins	11–13.29 mins	Under 11 mins
1500m	>45 mins	30–44.59 mins	24–29.59 mins	Under 24 mins
3000m	>100 mins	65–99.59 mins	50–64.59 mins	Under 50 mins
Functional Fitness (All)				
Pull-up	0	1–5	5–15	>15
Number of press-ups in 2 min	<15	15–29	30–79	>80
Number of burpees in 1 min	<15	15–24	25–39	>40
Standing jump	<2m	2–2.15m	2.16–2.44m	>2.45m
Elbow plank	0–60 secs	>60 secs	30-sec plank 4 x 15 secs 3 points of contact (3POC)	30-sec plank 4 x 15 secs 3 points of contact 2 x 15 secs 2 points of contact 30-sec plank

Female Performance Standards

Cardiovascular Fitness Activity (Pick 1 of 3)	Level 1	Level 2	Level 3	Paratrooper
Running / Rowing				
2.4km	>13.31 mins	11.30–13.30 mins	8.45–11.31 mins	Under 8.45 mins
10km	>65 mins	50–65 mins	42–50 mins	Under 42 mins
16km	>95 mins	85–95 mins	70–85 mins	Under 70 mins
Swimming				
750m	>20 mins	14.30–19.59 mins	12–14.29 mins	Under 12 mins
1500m	>45 mins	32–44.59 mins	26–31.59 mins	Under 26 mins
3000m	>100 mins	70–99.59 mins	54–69.59 mins	Under 54 mins
Functional Fitness (All)				
Pull-up	0	1–3	4–7	>8
Number of press-ups in 2 mins	0	1–14	15–35	>36
Number of burpees in 1 min	0	1–20	21–34	>35
Standing jump	<1.5m	1.5–1.64m	1.65–1.89m	>1.90m
Elbow plank	0–60 secs	>60 secs	30-sec plank 4 x 15 secs 3 points of contact (3POC)	30-sec plank 4 x 15 secs 3 points of contact 2 x 15 secs 2 points of contact 30-sec plank

FITNESS DRILLS

Just as paratroopers rely on drills to equip them for the battlefield, the PARA Fit training programmes also leverage **the power of drills to build instinctive patterns of activity, making fitness acquisition quicker and easier**. On the battlefield slick drills reign supreme and can be lifesaving; in fitness they amplify and embed your training regime. As we learnt in Chapter 1, the more instinctive we can make the execution of your training programme, the more successful you'll be.

Each of the programmes is based on a simple four-week repeating pattern – or a series of drills, comprised of some or all of the following:

- **Drill 1** warm-up;
- **Drill 2** mobility exercises;
- **Drill 3** circuit training;
- **Drill 4** cardio training;
- **Drill 5** cool down;
- **Drill 6** self-myofascial release (SMR)/foam rolling.

By focusing on a fixed number of functional movements and endurance activities you're able to master each pattern and focus on intensity and performance instead of perfecting new skills. By using benchmarks such as heart rate, resistance and your most recent max repetitions you are able to moderate intensity, so the programme adapts and evolves as your fitness improves.

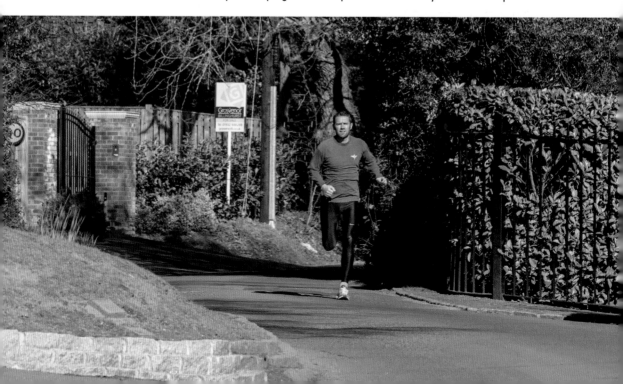

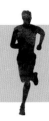

DRILL 1
WARM-UP

The warm-up is an essential component of a physical training session, which prepares you mentally and physically for the demands of training.

Each of the training sessions already has relevant muscle activation and mobility built into their design. So, all you need to do is 3–5 minutes of aerobic activity using one of the following: running, static cycling, rowing, skipping or the cross-trainer. My personal preference for running and cycling sessions is a gentle start, whereas for all strength sessions my staple is 5 minutes of either skipping or rowing.

Benefits of warm-up:
- reduces risk of injury;
- enhances performance;
- improves rate of training development;
- increases blood flow, delivering more oxygen to the working muscle;
- improves muscle strength and power.

Key points of warm-up:
- maximum 5 minutes in duration;
- targeted to specific training session activities;
- progressive in intensity, but must not adversely affect performance in main session;
- minimize transition period between end of warm-up and starting training activity to achieve maximum benefit.

WARM-UP EXERCISES
3–5-minute pulse raiser using one of the following exercises:
- running
- indoor cycling
- skipping
- running on the spot
- indoor rowing
- cross trainer

MOBILIZING MUSCLE GROUPS

We covered the importance of mobility both in training and in our daily lives in detail in Chapter 2. A dynamic warm-up, comprising mobility exercises that incorporate full range of movement (ROM) for the session's training activity, is now widely recognized as the optimum approach, after research demonstrated that static stretching offers little or no benefit.

After completing your 3–5-minute warm-up, prior to circuit training it's important you mobilize the relevant muscle groups before putting them under stress. Where relevant, each of the training sessions includes a sequence of 12 mobility exercises designed to prepare your body for the demands of the day. In the Boot Camp programme this sequence will help you adapt to your new regime and comprise the whole session two days per week.

Benefits of mobility exercises:
- reduces risk of injury;
- enhances performance;
- improves range of movement;
- increases motion control;
- improves muscle strength.

Key points of mobility exercises:
- targeted to specific training session activities;
- minimize transition period between end of warm-up and mobility exercises to achieve maximum benefit;
- 12-pattern sequence, holding each pose on each side of the body for maximum 30 seconds.

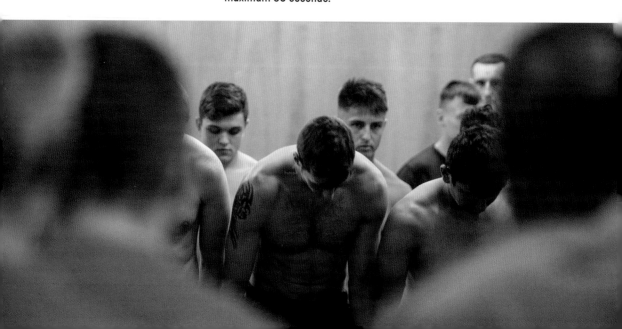

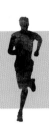

DRILL 2
MOBILITY EXERCISES

1. Warrior I

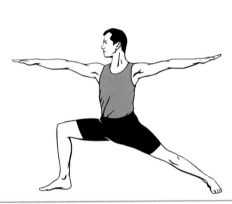

2. Warrior II

3. Lunge

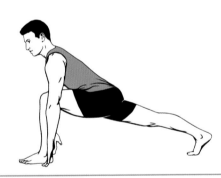

4. Lunge twist

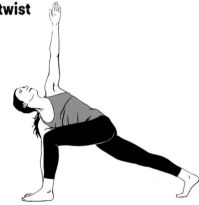

5. Pigeon pose

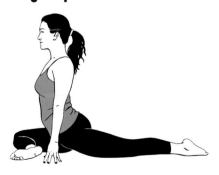

6. Downward dog

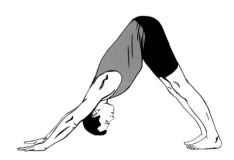

7. Upward dog

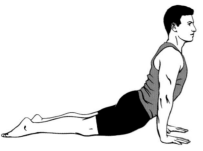

8. Cat pose

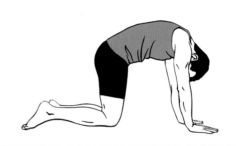

9. Cow pose

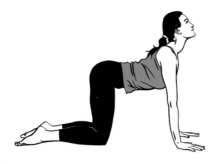

10. Child pose

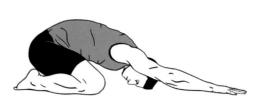

11. Bow pose

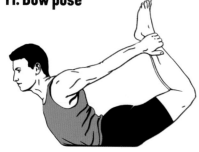

12. Reclining hero

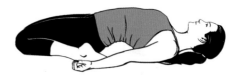

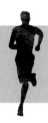

DRILL 3
CIRCUIT TRAINING

Circuit training is the name given to a group of strength exercises that are completed one after another, with each exercise being performed for a specified number of repetitions, or for a prescribed period of time, before moving on to the next exercise. It is an excellent way to improve all aspects of personal fitness. Circuit training has a number of advantages when compared with other forms of exercise:

- It develops both strength and muscular endurance at the same time.
- It can be tailored to most sports as well as to varying fitness and health levels.
- It can be conducted effectively without the use of specialized fitness equipment.

Even for someone new to training, it is easy to create a good circuit training session. The total number and type of circuit exercises performed during a training session can be changed to fit your ability, the time available for training, or your training goal. It is easy to tailor your session to a specific fitness goal, but a general circuit training session will normally include a circuit of exercises performed for a number of rotations. It is common to rest for a set period between each exercise. **Superset** is the term used to describe alternating between activities which focus on different muscle groups.

You can alter the number of repetitions you do of each exercise along with the total number of circuits you do, but as well as a warm-up and cool down, a session would typically include 4–8 incremental circuits, which are time or repetition based. In all of the PARA Fit programmes weight-based exercises are intended to be completed using 3 sets of 10 repetitions; and for non-weighted exercises, 3 sets of maximum repetitions in 30 seconds.

All of the training activities include **12 functional movement patterns**:

- **Bear crawl**
- **Bending pull**
- **Plank**
- **Bending push**
- **Standing jump**
- **Twist**
- **Burpees**
- **Vertical push**
- **Vertical pull**
- **Horizontal pull**
- **Squat**
- **Horizontal push**

By using compound movements that incorporate cohesive groups of different muscles, we are able to build function, strength and muscle growth concurrently, saving precious time, versus using exercises that isolate individual muscles. One major weakness of compound movements is their potential for injury, which we mitigate by using a small set of movements, investing heavily in form and increasing intensity gradually. Early on your best bet is to show your form and range of movement to a trained eye and seek their feedback; otherwise use YouTube and/or a mirror to assess yourself with a light load.

COMMON MOVEMENT PATTERNS

1. Bear crawl

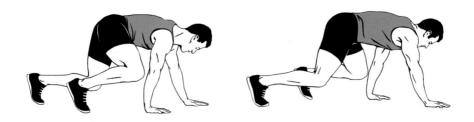

2. Plank variations

Arm plank

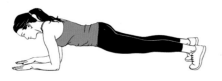

Elbow plank

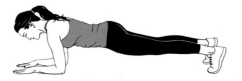

3 points of contact (POC)

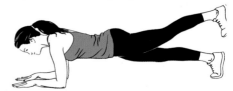

3. Standing jump

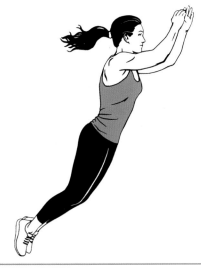

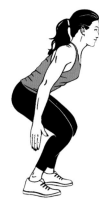

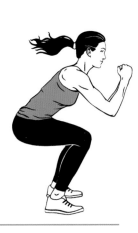

4. Burpees

* For safety, ensure a personal trainer or equivalent is present to help you with this exercise.

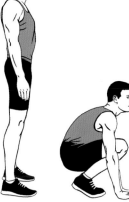

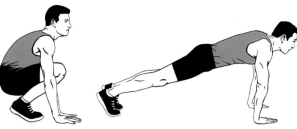

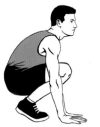

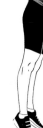

HOME DRILLS

1. Vertical pull

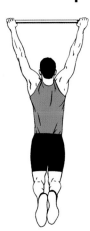

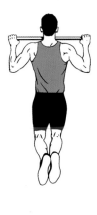

2. Squat

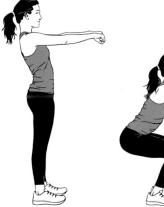

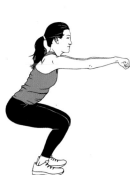

3. Bending pull/Romanian deadlift

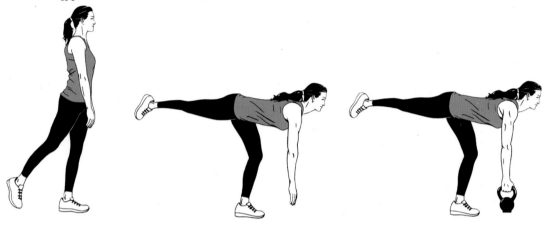

4. Bending push/sit-up

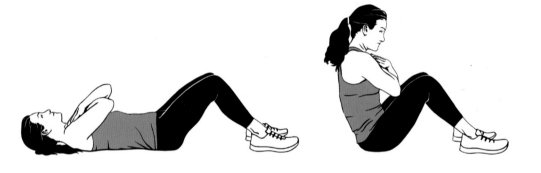

5. Twist

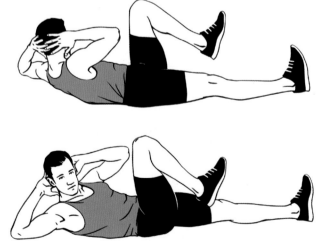

6. Vertical push

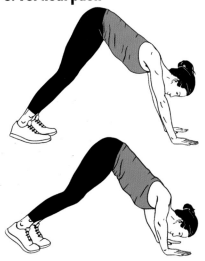
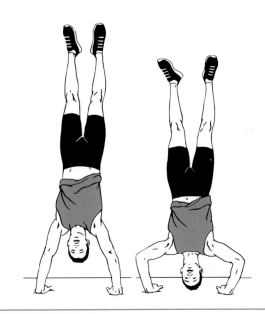

7. Horizontal pull

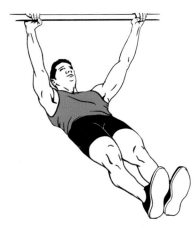
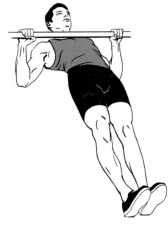

8. Horizontal push

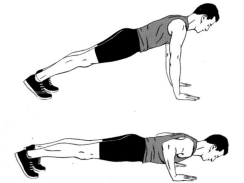
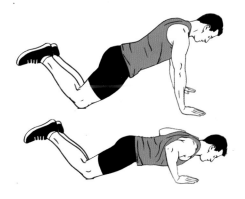

GYM DRILLS

1. Vertical pull

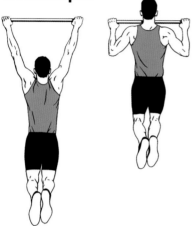

2. Squat

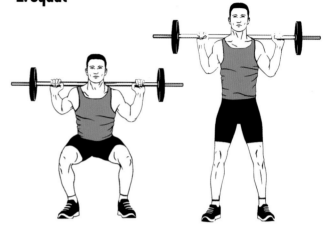

3. Bending pull/deadlift

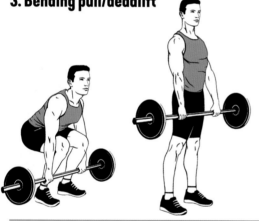

4. Bending push/sit-up

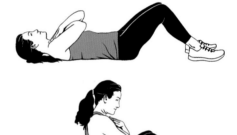

5. Twist

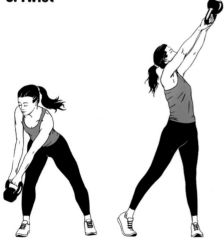

6. Vertical push/ military press

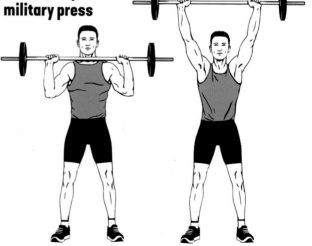

7. Horizontal pull/bent-over row

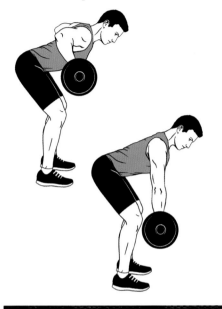

8. Horizontal push/bench press

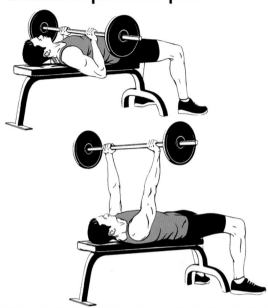

GAUGING WEIGHT-TRAINING INTENSITY

When building your own training programme, use the following planning guidelines to tailor your intensity and recovery to achieve your desired goal.

Objective	Perceived Effort	% of 1 Rep Max	Sets	Reps	Recovery Between Sets
Max strength	Hard/very hard	85–100	3–5	1–4	3–5 secs
Explosive strength	Moderately hard/very hard	80–95	3–5	1–5	3–5 secs
Muscular growth	Medium/moderately hard	60–80	3–5	6–10	30–60 secs
Muscular strength	Low/medium	30–60	3	10+	30–60 secs

All of the strength sessions in the training programmes are focused on promoting muscular growth at 70% effort. We use 3 sets of 10 reps for weights and 3x max reps in 30 seconds for no weights.

In both the PARA Fit and P Company programmes we use supersets to maximize training time efficiency, while ensuring adequate recovery for the resting muscle group.

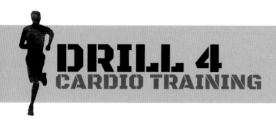

DRILL 4
CARDIO TRAINING

All training programmes include at least two days per week of cardio training. These sessions are designed for running, rowing or swimming. The heart rate (HR) guidance is geared to running, as max heart rate varies greatly between different activities, but the perceived effort levels detailed on page 98 should act as a consistent guide.

LIGHT ACTIVITY/ACTIVE RECOVERY (60% MAX HR)

These sessions are purposefully designed to be slow, to either acclimatize your body to training or aid recovery following intense training or competition. These sessions often feel too slow to be adding value, but play a vital role in the training process of stress, adaptation and recovery.

Light activity sessions feature in the Boot Camp programme to help build a stable foundation of fitness. Recovery sessions feature in the de-load week of the other programmes to help your body adapt to and recover from three weeks of cumulative training load.

FUEL-EFFICIENCY TRAINING (70% MAX HR)

Fuel-efficiency training involves training at a level well below your aerobic threshold. Its purpose is to improve your body's ability to use fat stores as an energy source. These sessions often feel slow and a little boring but are your best means of teaching your body to burn fat instead of carbohydrates, which is relevant for any training session or competition greater than two hours. We use fuel-efficiency sessions in the Fighting Fit programme and every week in the Paratrooper programmes. For these sessions to be effective, they are best done first thing in the morning on an empty stomach, without consuming any food during the session.

THRESHOLD TRAINING (85% MAX HR)

Threshold, or tempo, training, as the name suggests, involves training at your aerobic threshold (as fast as possible aerobically) for a continuous period. This type of training session works by gradually increasing the pace and duration at which your body can deal with the lactic acid produced during exertion. It is best to progress slowly into tempo running by either starting slowly or breaking your run into phases – like an interval session, but with less rest time between the interval paces. We use threshold training in the Fighting Fit, Paratrooper and P Company programmes.

INTERVAL TRAINING (90% MAX HR)

Interval training, as the name suggests, involves training at a specific intensity for a sustained period, followed by a rest, followed by repeating this process a number of times. Interval training is an extremely effective method of training and works by overloading the body and educating it on what it feels like to run/cycle/swim/row quicker than it is used to. Interval sessions can be measured by time or distance, and hill reps are a type of interval training that use gradient instead of speed to increase intensity. Interval sessions can be measured by time or distance. If you're new to interval training, be warned: it hurts! The trick is to build up slowly. But take comfort that with interval training you are igniting your mental resilience while propelling your fitness. We will use interval training in all but the Boot Camp programme.

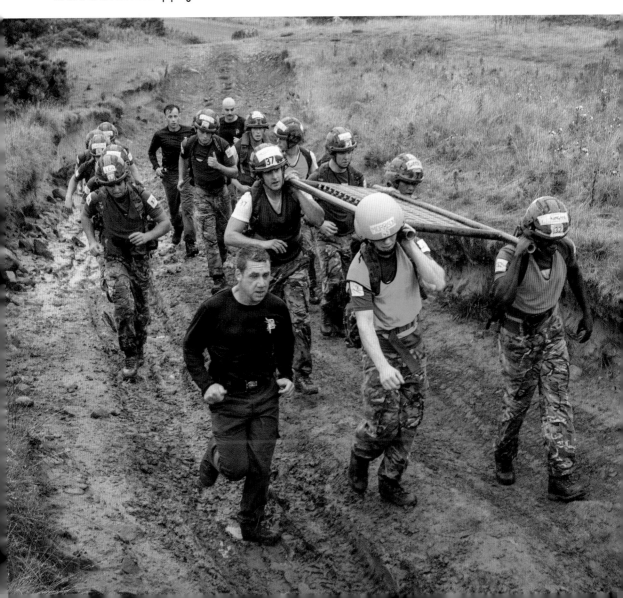

CARDIO TRAINING EFFORT

The intensity of training determines not only the effort level but the energy source that fuels the activity. Lower exertion is fuelled by body fat; as effort intensifies it becomes fuelled increasingly from glycogen stores (carbohydrates). The table below illustrates the perceived effort and various max heart rate levels, to aid those not training with a fitness watch that measures HR.

Effort	Description	% of Maximum Heart Rate*
No exertion	Little to no movement	20
Extremely light	Minimal movement	30
Very light	Comfortable, increased breathing	50
Light/recovery	Minimal sweating, can talk easily	60
Moderate	Slight breathlessness, can talk	70
Moderately hard	Increased sweating, able to hold conversation with difficulty	80
Hard	Sweating, able to push and still maintain correct form	85
Very hard	Can maintain pace for a short time period	90
Extremely hard	Difficulty breathing, near muscular exhaustion	100
Maximum	Stop exercising, total exhaustion	

* Maximum heart rate can be estimated by using 220 minus age (10–12% variance).

ENERGY SYSTEMS

For those with a technical interest... During training the body deploys three main energy systems to fuel activity dependent on the intensity. While there are many expressions of energy output, the duration and intensity (e.g. a 50m sprint vs a half-marathon) govern which energy system is used. All are available and are initiated at the outset of activity. The primary determiner of which system(s) is/are used is the effort expended.

ATP system – burst duration, maximal effort.

ATP (adenosine triphosphate) is a molecule that is the primary energy source used by muscles for contraction. The ATP-PC energy (or Phosphogen) system allows for approximately 12 seconds of maximum effort. It is immediate and requires no oxygen. Estimates suggest that the ATP-PC system creates energy at 36 calories per minute. It is used for high-power, short duration bursts such as a short sprint, or maximum weight repetition.

Glycotic system – short duration, sub-maximal effort.

The glycotic system initiates after the ATP-PC is depleted, and estimates indicate that it produces 16 calories per minute. The glycotic system is fuelled by dietary carbohydrates circulating in the blood or stored as glycogen in muscles of the liver. Depending on intensity it is further categorized as fast glycosis (quick decline at approximately 1 minute) or slow glycosis (slower decline >1 minute). This energy system is utilized for activities such as the 400m hurdles or a 2km row.

Oxidative system – low power, long duration.

The oxidative system is always active and is the body's recovery mechanism. It is the primary energy source for low-power, long-duration activities. Research suggest that the oxidative system generates 10 calories per minute. The oxidative system is fuelled by either carbohydrates, of which the body stores approximately 2,000 calories in glycogen in the blood, muscles and liver, or fat, which it has in vast supply from the body's fat tissue. Because fat takes more time to break down than glycogen, more oxygen is needed for combustion. The more intense the exertion, the more the oxidative system relies on carbohydrates, which deplete more quickly. In extended activities, the body may also convert protein to energy as the fuel of last resort, albeit less efficiently and at a slower rate than carbohydrates.

While ATP-PC and glycotic training sessions burn more calories during and after the workouts, making them more efficient training sessions from an output perspective, recovery is exclusively aerobic. Training the oxidative system improves aerobic capacity, recovery and durability and provides more oxygen and nutrients to the tissues. It is estimated that the ATP-PC and glycotic systems can be improved by 20%, and oxidative by 50%, through targeted training and optimal nutrition. However, genetics also play a key part. Muscle fibre composition is unalterable, potentially predisposing you to endurance- (type 1 fibres) or strength- (type 2 fibres) based activities which play to your genetic strengths. Notwithstanding this, while the composition should vary for each sport, continually training different energy systems encourages your body to adapt and is critical to performance across all sports.

Across the four training programmes we toggle between ATP and glycotic systems for the circuit training sessions, and glycotic and oxidative systems for the cardio sessions.

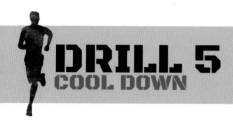

DRILL 5
COOL DOWN

The cool down is an integral part of every physical training session, often overlooked on the false assumption that the hardest part of the session is the most important part. Physical activity results in tighter muscles and tendons, reducing range of movement (ROM) and increasing risk of injury. A well-designed cool down enhances training adaptation by promoting recovery. Such a session includes mobilizing joints, lengthening muscles and tendons, and ultimately returning the body to its resting state. All cool downs should be focused on the muscles used during the session's activity.

All programmes include six of the 12 mobility exercises used at the start of each session as a cool down, both reinforcing correct form through repetition and maximizing the power of drills to effectively cool down the body's major muscle groups.

Benefits of cool down:
- helps return the body to its normal resting state;
- reduces potential of developing delayed onset muscle soreness (DOMS);
- reduces potential for dizziness and fainting;
- reduces adrenaline in blood;
- normalizes muscle length and tension;
- offers chance to reflect on session;
- helps you be better prepared for next session;
- aids in removal of waste products such as lactic acid.

Key points of cool down:
- circa 5 minutes in duration;
- targeted to specific training session activities;
- hold positions for 30 seconds.

COOL DOWN EXERCISES

1. Lunge twist (each side)

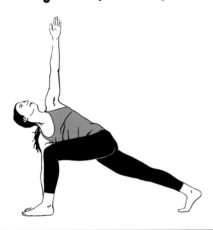

2. Downward dog

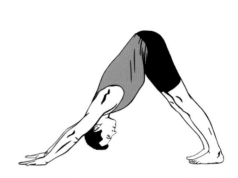

3. Upward dog

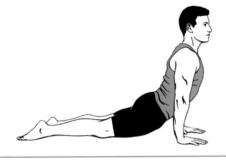

4. Cat pose

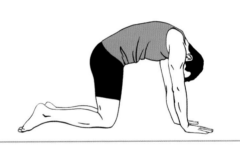

5. Child pose

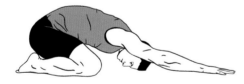

6. Reclining hero

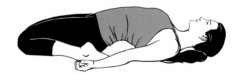

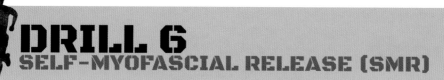

DRILL 6
SELF-MYOFASCIAL RELEASE (SMR)

SMR/foam rolling is a form of self-massage using a foam roller or similar object instead of a therapist. The 14 exercises are a mix of static trigger point (sore, tight area) and rolling exercises. The process targets tightness in soft tissues to help recovery and performance. We use SMR extensively across all the programmes to promote mobility and recovery between sessions.

Benefits of SMR:
- breaks down scar tissue and stickiness/adhesions connecting muscles and connective tissues;
- improves acute flexibility/mobility and thereby reduces risk of injury;
- cheaper than massage.

Key points of SMR:
- uses body weight to apply focused pressure to areas of muscular and tendon tightness;
- can be used on all fleshy parts on body – not joints;
- when a trigger point is felt, hold and apply pressure for 10 seconds, then carry on rolling the area;
- aim for three trigger points in each major muscle group.

SMR EXERCISES
1. Sole of foot (static)   2. Calf muscle

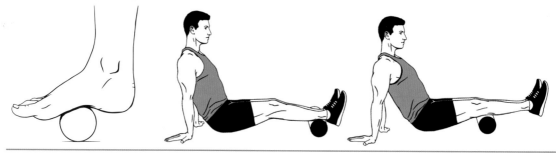

3. Tibia anterior

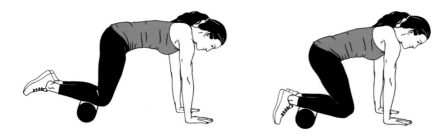

4. Hamstring

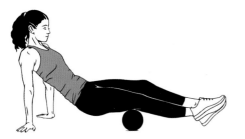 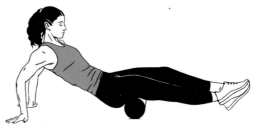

5. Inner thigh (static)

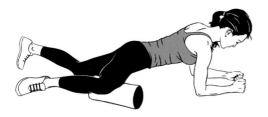

6. Hip flexor & quad (static)

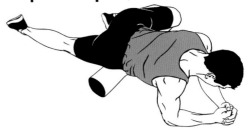

7. Iliotibial band (ITB)

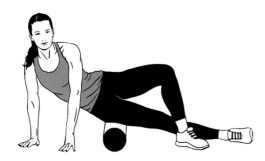 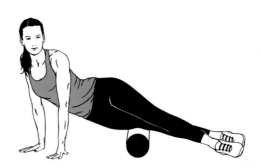

8. Glutes

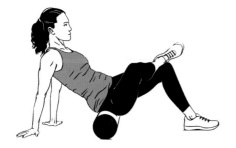

9. Lower back

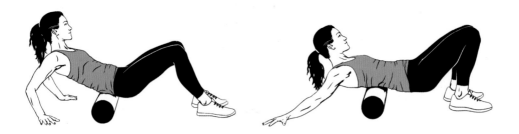

10. Lats dorsi (Lats)

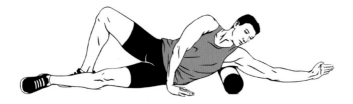

11. Pecs (static)

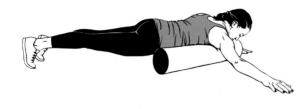

12. Traps (static)

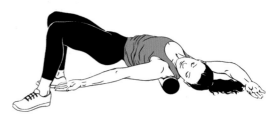

13. Deltoids (static)

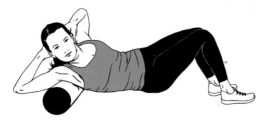

14. Neck (static)

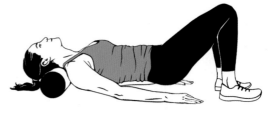

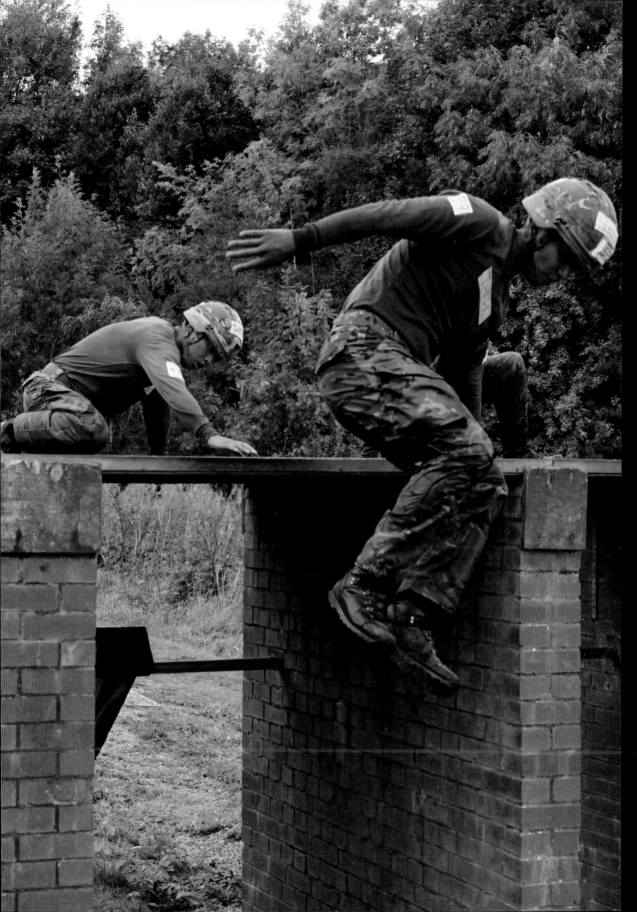

WEEK 1 (LOAD)

MONDAY

DRILL 1: Warm-Up: 3–5 mins cardio
DRILL 2: Mobility: 12-Exercise Sequence (2 x 30 secs each side)
Function Assessment: Overhead squat • Inline lunge • Hurdle step • Shoulder mobility • Active straight leg raise • Trunk stability push-up • Rotary stability
Cardio Assessment: (1 of 3) • Run or row 2.4km • Swim 750m
DRILL 3: Circuit Training: (max) Standing jump • Press-up (modified) – 2 mins • Arm plank *(handwritten: CDo three times each — for 30 reps)*
DRILL 5: Cool Down: 6-Exercise Sequence (30 secs each)

29 Jan

TUESDAY

Rest

27 Jan

WEDNESDAY

DRILL 1: Warm-Up: 3–5 mins cardio
DRILL 2: Mobility: 12-Exercise Sequence (2 x 30 secs each side)
DRILL 4: Cardio: Light activity (run/swim/cycle) 30 mins @ 60% max HR
DRILL 5: Cool Down: 6-Exercise Sequence (30 secs each)

30 Jan

THURSDAY

DRILL 1: Warm-Up: 3–5 mins cardio
DRILL 2: Mobility: 12-Exercise Sequence (4 x 30 secs each side)

29 Jan

FRIDAY

DRILL 6: SMR: (1 min each) Glutes • Lower back • Lats • Pecs • Traps • Deltoids • Neck

5 Jan

SATURDAY

DRILL 1: Warm-Up: 3–5 mins cardio
DRILL 2: Mobility: 12-Exercise Sequence (2 x 30 secs each side)
DRILL 4: Cardio: Light activity (run/swim/row) 30 mins @ 60% max HR
DRILL 5: Cool Down: 6-Exercise Sequence (30 secs each)

24 Jan

SUNDAY

DRILL 6: SMR: 14-Exercise Sequence (1 min each) as follows: Sole of foot • Calf muscle • Tibia anterior • Hamstring • Inner thigh • Hip flexor & quad • ITB • Glutes • Lower back • Lats • Pecs • Traps • Deltoids • Neck

26 Jan

WEEK 2 (LOAD)

MONDAY

DRILL 1: Warm-Up: 3–5 mins cardio
DRILL 2: Mobility: 12-Exercise Sequence (4 x 30 secs each side)

TUESDAY

DRILL 6: SMR: (1 min each) Sole of foot • Calf muscle • Tibia anterior • Hamstring • Inner thigh • Hip flexor & quad • ITB

WEDNESDAY

DRILL 1: Warm-Up: 3–5 mins cardio
DRILL 2: Mobility: 12-Exercise Sequence (2 x 30 secs each side)
DRILL 4: Cardio: Light activity (run/swim/row) 30 mins @ 60% max HR
DRILL 5: Cool Down: 6-Exercise Sequence (30 secs each)

THURSDAY

DRILL 1: Warm-Up: 3–5 mins cardio
DRILL 2: Mobility: 12-Exercise Sequence (4 x 30 secs each side)

FRIDAY

DRILL 6: SMR: (1 min each) Glutes • Lower back • Lats • Pecs • Traps • Deltoids • Neck

SATURDAY

DRILL 1: Warm-Up: 3–5 mins cardio
DRILL 2: Mobility: 12-Exercise Sequence (2 x 30 secs each side)
DRILL 4: Cardio: Light activity (run/swim/row) 30 mins @ 60% max HR
DRILL 5: Cool Down: 6-Exercise Sequence (30 secs each)

SUNDAY

DRILL 6: SMR: 14-Exercise Sequence (1 min each) as follows: (1 min each) Sole of foot • Calf muscle • Tibia anterior • Hamstring • Inner thigh • Hip flexor & quad • ITB • Glutes • Lower back • Lats • Pecs • Traps • Deltoids • Neck

LEVEL 1: BOOT CAMP PROGRAMME

MONDAY

DRILL 1: Warm-Up: 3–5 mins cardio
DRILL 2: Mobility: 12-Exercise Sequence (4 x 30 secs each side)

TUESDAY

DRILL 6: SMR: (1 min each) Sole of foot • Calf muscle • Tibia anterior • Hamstring • Inner thigh • Hip flexor & quad • ITB

WEDNESDAY

DRILL 1: Warm-Up: 3–5 mins cardio
DRILL 2: Mobility: 12-Exercise Sequence (2 x 30 secs each side)
DRILL 4: Cardio: Light activity (run/swim/row) 30 mins @ 60% max HR
DRILL 5: Cool Down: 6-Exercise Sequence (30 secs each)

THURSDAY

DRILL 1: Warm-Up: 3–5 mins cardio
DRILL 2: Mobility: 12-Exercise Sequence (4 x 30 secs each side)

FRIDAY

DRILL 6: SMR: (1 min each) Glutes • Lower back
• Lats • Pecs • Traps • Deltoids • Neck

SATURDAY

DRILL 1: Warm-Up: 3–5 mins cardio
DRILL 2: Mobility: 12-Exercise Sequence (2 x 30 secs each side)
DRILL 4: Cardio: Light activity (run/swim/row) 30 mins @ 60% max HR
DRILL 5: Cool Down: 6-Exercise Sequence (30 secs each)

SUNDAY

DRILL 6: SMR: 14-Exercise Sequence (1 min each) as follows: (1 min each) Sole of foot • Calf muscle • Tibia anterior • Hamstring • Inner thigh • Hip flexor & quad • ITB • Glutes • Lower back • Lats • Pecs • Traps • Deltoids • Neck

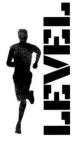

WEEK 4 (DE-LOAD)

MONDAY

DRILL 1: Warm-Up: 3–5 mins cardio
DRILL 2: Mobility: 12-Exercise Sequence (4 x 30 secs each side)

TUESDAY

DRILL 6: SMR: (1 min each) Sole of foot • Calf muscle • Tibia anterior • Hamstring • Inner thigh • Hip flexor & quad • ITB

WEDNESDAY

DRILL 1: Warm-Up: 3–5 mins cardio
DRILL 2: Mobility: 12-Exercise Sequence (2 x 30 secs each side)
DRILL 4: Cardio: Light activity (run/swim/row) 30 mins @ 60% max HR
DRILL 5: Cool Down: 6-Exercise Sequence (30 secs each)

THURSDAY

DRILL 1: Warm-Up: 3–5 mins cardio
DRILL 2: Mobility: 12-Exercise Sequence (4 x 30 secs each side)

FRIDAY

DRILL 6: SMR: (1 min each) Glutes • Lower back • Lats • Pecs • Traps • Deltoids • Neck

SATURDAY

DRILL 1: Warm-Up: 3–5 mins cardio
DRILL 2: Mobility: 12-Exercise Sequence (2 x 30 secs each side)
DRILL 4: Cardio: Light activity (run/swim/row) 30 mins @ 60% max HR
DRILL 5: Cool Down: 6-Exercise Sequence (30 secs each)

SUNDAY

DRILL 6: SMR: 14-Exercise Sequence (1 min each) as follows: (1 min each) Sole of foot • Calf muscle • Tibia anterior • Hamstring • Inner thigh • Hip flexor & quad • ITB • Glutes • Lower back • Lats • Pecs • Traps • Deltoids • Neck

LEVEL 2: FIGHTING FIT PROGRAMME

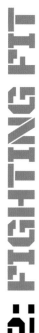

MONDAY

DRILL 1: Warm-Up: 3–5 mins cardio
DRILL 2: Mobility: 12-Exercise Sequence (2 x 30 secs each side)
Function Assessment: Overhead squat • Inline lunge • Hurdle step
• Shoulder mobility • Active straight leg raise • Trunk stability push-up
• Rotary stability
Cardio Assessment: (1 of 3) Run or row 2.4km • Swim 750m
DRILL 3: Circuit Training: (max) Pull-up • Standing jump • Press-up – 2
mins • Elbow plank • Burpees – 1 min
DRILL 5: Cool Down: 6-Exercise Sequence (30 secs each)

TUESDAY

Rest

WEDNESDAY

DRILL 1: Warm-Up: 3–5 mins cardio
DRILL 2: Mobility: 12-Exercise Sequence (2 x 30 secs each side)
DRILL 4: Cardio: Threshold (run/row/swim/row) 20 mins @ 85% max HR
• 3-min walk at end
DRILL 5: Cool Down: 6-Exercise Sequence (30 secs each)

THURSDAY

DRILL 1: Warm-Up: 3–5 mins cardio
DRILL 2: Mobility: 12-Exercise Sequence (2 x 30 secs each side)
DRILL 3: Circuit Training: 3 x (30 secs or 10 reps) Twist (both sides) •
Vertical push • Horizontal pull • Horizontal push • Burpees • (1-min rest
between sets)
DRILL 5: Cool Down: 6-Exercise Sequence (30 secs each)

FRIDAY

Rest

SATURDAY

DRILL 1: Warm-Up: 3–5 mins cardio
DRILL 2: Mobility: 12-Exercise Sequence (2 x 30 secs each side)
DRILL 4: Cardio: Fuel Efficiency (run/swim/cycle) 30 mins @ 70% max HR
DRILL 5: Cool Down: 6-Exercise Sequence (30 secs each)

SUNDAY

DRILL 6: SMR: 14-Exercise Sequence (1 min each) as follows: (1 min each)
Sole of foot • Calf muscle • Tibia anterior • Hamstring • Inner thigh • Hip flexor
& quad • ITB • Glutes • Lower back • Lats • Pecs • Traps • Deltoids • Neck

WEEK 2 (LOAD)

MONDAY

DRILL 1: Warm-Up: 3–5 mins cardio
DRILL 2: Mobility: 12-Exercise Sequence (2 x 30 secs each side)
DRILL 3: Circuit Training: 3 x (30 secs or 10 reps) Vertical pull • Squat •
Bending pull • Bending push • Elbow plank • (1 min rest between sets)
DRILL 5: Cool Down: 6-Exercise Sequence (30 secs each)

TUESDAY

DRILL 1: Warm-Up: 3–5 mins cardio
DRILL 2: Mobility: 12-Exercise Sequence (2 x 30 secs each side)
DRILL 4: Cardio: Fuel Efficiency (run/swim/row) 30 mins @ 70% max HR •
No food 8 hrs before or during session • 3-min walk at end
DRILL 5: Cool Down: 6-Exercise Sequence (30 secs each)

WEDNESDAY

DRILL 1: Warm-Up: 3–5 mins cardio
DRILL 2: Mobility: 12-Exercise Sequence (2 x 30 secs each side)
DRILL 4: Cardio: Intervals (run/swim/row) 8 x 2 mins @ 80% max HR
(3-min rest between intervals) • 3-min walk at end
DRILL 5: Cool Down: 6-Exercise Sequence (30 secs each)

THURSDAY

DRILL 1: Warm-Up: 3–5 mins cardio
DRILL 2: Mobility: 12-Exercise Sequence (2 x 30 secs each side)
DRILL 3: Circuit Training: 3 x (30 secs or 10 reps) • Twist (both sides) •
Vertical push • Horizontal pull • Horizontal push • Burpees • (1-min rest
between sets)
DRILL 5: Cool Down: 6-Exercise Sequence (30 secs each)

FRIDAY

Rest

SATURDAY

DRILL 1: Warm-Up: 3–5 mins cardio
DRILL 2: Mobility: 12-Exercise Sequence (2 x 30 secs each side)
DRILL 4: Cardio: Fuel Efficiency (run/swim/cycle) 30 mins @ 70% max HR
DRILL 5: Cool Down: 6-Exercise Sequence (30 secs each)

SUNDAY

DRILL 6: SMR: 14-Exercise Sequence (1 min each) as follows: Sole of foot
• Calf muscle • Tibia anterior • Hamstring • Inner thigh • Hip flexor & quad
• ITB • Glutes • Lower back • Lats • Pecs • Traps • Deltoids • Neck

LEVEL 2: FIGHTING FIT PROGRAMME

MONDAY

DRILL 1: Warm-Up: 3–5 mins cardio
DRILL 2: Mobility: 12-Exercise Sequence (2 x 30 secs each side)
DRILL 3: Circuit Training: 3 x (30 secs or 10 reps) • Vertical pull • Squat • Bending pull • Bending push • Elbow plank • (1-min rest between sets)
DRILL 5: Cool Down: 6-Exercise Sequence (30 secs each)

TUESDAY

DRILL 1: Warm-Up: 3–5 mins cardio
DRILL 2: Mobility: 12-Exercise Sequence (2 x 30 secs each side)
DRILL 4: Cardio: Fuel Efficiency (run/swim/row) 30 mins @ 70% max HR • No food 8 hrs before or during session • 3-min walk at end
DRILL 5: Cool Down: 6-Exercise Sequence (30 secs each)

WEDNESDAY

DRILL 1: Warm-Up: 3–5 mins cardio
DRILL 2: Mobility: 12-Exercise Sequence (2 x 30 secs each side)
DRILL 4: Cardio: Intervals (run/swim/row) 5 x 3 mins @ 85% max HR (3-min rest between intervals) • 3-min walk at end
DRILL 5: Cool Down: 6-Exercise Sequence (30 secs each)

THURSDAY

DRILL 1: Warm-Up: 3–5 mins cardio
DRILL 2: Mobility: 12-Exercise Sequence (2 x 30 secs each side)
DRILL 3: Circuit Training: 3 x (30 secs or 10 reps) • Twist (both sides) • Vertical push • Horizontal pull • Horizontal push • Burpees • (1-min rest between sets)
DRILL 5: Cool Down: 6-Exercise Sequence (30 secs each)

FRIDAY

Rest

SATURDAY

DRILL 1: Warm-Up: 3–5 mins cardio
DRILL 2: Mobility: 12-Exercise Sequence (2 x 30 secs each side)
DRILL 4: Cardio: Fuel Efficiency (run/swim/cycle) 30 mins @ 70% max HR
DRILL 5: Cool Down: 6-Exercise Sequence (30 secs each)

SUNDAY

DRILL 6: SMR: 14-Exercise Sequence (1 min each) as follows: Sole of foot • Calf muscle • Tibia anterior • Hamstring • Inner thigh • Hip flexor & quad • ITB • Glutes • Lower back • Lats • Pecs • Traps • Deltoids • Neck

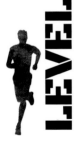

WEEK 4 (DE-LOAD)

MONDAY

DRILL 1: **Warm-Up:** 3–5 mins cardio
DRILL 2: **Mobility:** 12-Exercise Sequence (2 x 30 secs each side)
DRILL 3: **Circuit Training:** 3 x (30 secs or 10 reps) • Vertical pull • Squat •
Bending pull • Bending push • Elbow plank • (1-min rest between sets)
DRILL 5: **Cool Down:** 6-Exercise Sequence (30 secs each)

TUESDAY

DRILL 1: **Warm-Up:** 3–5 mins cardio
DRILL 2: **Mobility:** 12-Exercise Sequence (2 x 30 secs each side)
DRILL 4: **Cardio:** Fuel Efficiency (run/swim/row) 30 mins @ 70% max HR
• No food 8 hrs before or during session • 3-min walk at end
DRILL 5: **Cool Down:** 6-Exercise Sequence (30 secs each)

WEDNESDAY

DRILL 1: **Warm-Up:** 3–5 mins cardio
DRILL 2: **Mobility:** 12-Exercise Sequence (2 x 30 secs each side)
DRILL 4: **Cardio:** Recovery (run/swim/row) 30 mins @ 60% max HR
DRILL 5: **Cool Down:** 6-Exercise Sequence (30 secs each)

THURSDAY

DRILL 1: **Warm-Up:** 3–5 mins cardio
DRILL 2: **Mobility:** 12-Exercise Sequence (2 x 30 secs each side)
DRILL 3: **Circuit Training:** 3 x (30 secs or 10 reps) • Twist (both sides) •
Vertical push • Horizontal pull • Horizontal push • Burpees • (1-min rest
between sets)
DRILL 5: **Cool Down:** 6-Exercise Sequence (30 secs each)

FRIDAY

Rest

SATURDAY

DRILL 1: **Warm-Up:** 3–5 mins cardio
DRILL 2: **Mobility:** 12-Exercise Sequence (2 x 30 secs each side)
DRILL 4: **Cardio:** Fuel Efficiency (run/swim/cycle) 30 mins @ 70% max HR
DRILL 5: **Cool Down:** 6-Exercise Sequence (30 secs each)

SUNDAY

DRILL 6: **SMR:** 14-Exercise Sequence (1 min each) as follows: Sole of foot
• Calf muscle • Tibia anterior • Hamstring • Inner thigh • Hip flexor & quad
• ITB • Glutes • Lower back • Lats • Pecs • Traps • Deltoids • Neck

LEVEL 3: PARA FIT PROGRAMME

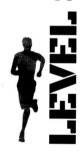

MONDAY

DRILL 1: Warm-Up: 3–5 mins cardio
DRILL 2: Mobility: 12-Exercise Sequence (2 x 30 secs each side)
Function Assessment: As previous programmes
Cardio Assessment: (1 of 4) Run or row 2.4km • Cycle 20km • Swim 750m
DRILL 3: Circuit Training: (max) • Pull-up • Standing jump • Press-up – 2 mins • Plank 3POC • Burpees – 1 min
DRILL 5: Cool Down: 6-Exercise Sequence (30 secs each)

TUESDAY

DRILL 6: SMR: 14-Exercise Sequence (1 min each)

WEDNESDAY

DRILL 1: Warm-Up: 3–5 mins cardio
DRILL 2: Mobility: 12-Exercise Sequence (2 x 30 secs each side)
DRILL 4: Cardio: Fuel Efficiency (run/swim/cycle) 30 mins @ 70% max HR
DRILL 5: Cool Down: 6-Exercise Sequence (30 secs each)

THURSDAY

DRILL 1: Warm-Up: 3–5 mins cardio
DRILL 2: Mobility: 12-Exercise Sequence (2 x 30 secs each side)
DRILL 3: Circuit Training: 3 x (30 secs or 10 reps) Superset • Twist (both sides)/vertical push • Horizontal pull/horizontal push • Vertical pull/squat • Bending pull/bending push • Plank (3POC)/burpees • Bear crawl
DRILL 5: Cool Down: 6-Exercise Sequence (30 secs each)

FRIDAY

DRILL 1: Warm-Up: 3–5 mins cardio
DRILL 2: Mobility: 12-Exercise Sequence (2 x 30 secs each side)
DRILL 4: Cardio: Light activity (run/walk/swim/cycle) 30 mins @ 60% max HR
DRILL 5: Cool Down: 6-Exercise Sequence (30 secs each)

SATURDAY

DRILL 1: Warm-Up: 3–5 mins cardio
DRILL 2: Mobility: 12-Exercise Sequence (2 x 30 secs each side)
DRILL 4: Cardio: Threshold (run/swim/row) 20 mins @ 85% max HR • 3-min walk at end
DRILL 5: Cool Down: 6-Exercise Sequence (30 secs each)

SUNDAY

DRILL 6: SMR: 14-Exercise Sequence (1 min each)

WEEK 2 (LOAD)

MONDAY

DRILL 1: Warm-Up: 3–5 mins cardio
DRILL 2: Mobility: 12-Exercise Sequence (2 x 30 secs each side)
DRILL 3: Circuit Training: 3 x (30 secs or 10 reps) Superset • Twist (both sides)/vertical push • Horizontal pull/horizontal push • Vertical pull/squat • Bending pull/bending push • Plank (3POC)/burpees • Bear crawl
DRILL 5: Cool Down: 6-Exercise Sequence (30 secs each)

TUESDAY

DRILL 1: Warm-Up: 3–5 mins cardio
DRILL 2: Mobility: 12-Exercise Sequence (2 x 30 secs each side)
DRILL 4: Cardio: Intervals (run/swim/row) 8 x 2 mins @ 90% max HR (3-min rest between intervals) • 3-min walk at end
DRILL 5: Cool Down: 6-Exercise Sequence (30 secs each)

WEDNESDAY

DRILL 1: Warm-Up: 3–5 mins cardio
DRILL 4: Cardio: Fuel efficiency (run/swim/row) 50 mins @ 70% max HR • No food 8 hrs before or during session • 3-min walk at end
DRILL 5: Cool Down: 6-Exercise Sequence (30 secs each)

THURSDAY

DRILL 1: Warm-Up: 3–5 mins cardio
DRILL 2: Mobility: 12-Exercise Sequence (2 x 30 secs each side)
DRILL 3: Circuit Training: As Monday: 3 x (30 secs or 10 reps)
DRILL 5: Cool Down: 6-Exercise Sequence (30 secs each)

FRIDAY

DRILL 1: Warm-Up: 3–5 mins cardio
DRILL 2: Mobility: 12-Exercise Sequence (2 x 30 secs each side)
DRILL 4: Cardio: Intervals (run/swim/row) 5 x 5 mins @ 85% max HR (3-min rest between intervals) • 3-min walk at end
DRILL 5: Cool Down: 6-Exercise Sequence (30 secs each)

SATURDAY

DRILL 1: Warm-Up: 3–5 mins cardio
DRILL 2: Mobility: 12-Exercise Sequence (2 x 30 secs each side)
DRILL 4: Cardio: Threshold (run/swim/row) 20 mins @ 85% max HR • 3-min walk at end
DRILL 5: Cool Down: 6-Exercise Sequence (30 secs each)

SUNDAY

DRILL 6: SMR: 14-Exercise Sequence (1 min each)

LEVEL 3: PARA FIT PROGRAMME

MONDAY

DRILL 1: **Warm-Up:** 3–5 mins cardio
DRILL 2: **Mobility:** 12-Exercise Sequence (2 x 30 secs each side)
DRILL 3: **Circuit Training:** 3 x (30 secs or 10 reps) Superset • Twist (both sides)/vertical push • Horizontal pull/horizontal push • Vertical pull/squat • Bending pull/bending push • Plank (3POC)/burpees • Bear crawl
DRILL 5: **Cool Down:** 6-Exercise Sequence (30 secs each)

TUESDAY

DRILL 1: **Warm-Up:** 3–5 mins cardio
DRILL 2: **Mobility:** 12-Exercise Sequence (2 x 30 secs each side)
DRILL 4: **Cardio:** Intervals (run/swim/row) 8 x 2 mins @ 90% max HR (3-min rest between intervals) • 3-min walk at end
DRILL 5: **Cool Down:** 6-Exercise Sequence (30 secs each)

WEDNESDAY

DRILL 1: **Warm-Up:** 3–5 mins cardio
DRILL 4: **Cardio:** Fuel Efficiency (run/swim/row) 50 mins @ 70% max HR • No food 8 hrs before or during session • 3-min walk at end
DRILL 5: **Cool Down:** 6-Exercise Sequence (30 secs each

THURSDAY

DRILL 1: **Warm-Up:** 3–5 mins cardio
DRILL 2: **Mobility:** 12-Exercise Sequence (2 x 30 secs each side)
DRILL 3: **Circuit Training:** As Monday: 3 x (30 secs or 10 reps)
DRILL 5: **Cool Down:** 6-Exercise Sequence (30 secs each)

FRIDAY

DRILL 1: **Warm-Up:** 3–5 mins cardio
DRILL 2: **Mobility:** 12-Exercise Sequence (2 x 30 secs each side)
DRILL 4: **Cardio:** Intervals (run/swim/row) 5 x 5 mins @ 85% max HR (3-min rest between intervals) • 3-min walk at end
DRILL 5: **Cool Down:** 6-Exercise Sequence (30 secs each)

SATURDAY

DRILL 1: **Warm-Up:** 3–5 mins cardio
DRILL 2: **Mobility:** 12-Exercise Sequence (2 x 30 secs each side)
DRILL 4: **Cardio:** Threshold (run/swim/row) 20 mins @ 85% max HR • 3-min walk at end
DRILL 5: **Cool down:** 6-Exercise Sequence (30 secs each)

SUNDAY

DRILL 6: **SMR:** 14-Exercise Sequence (1 min each)

WEEK 4 (DE-LOAD)

MONDAY

DRILL 1: Warm-Up: 3–5 mins cardio
DRILL 2: Mobility: 12-Exercise Sequence (2 x 30 secs each side)
DRILL 3: Circuit Training: 3 x (30 secs or 10 reps) Superset • Twist (both sides)/vertical push • Horizontal pull/horizontal push • Vertical pull/squat • Bending pull/bending push • Plank (3POC)/burpees • Bear crawl
DRILL 5: Cool Down: 6-Exercise Sequence (30 secs each)

TUESDAY

DRILL 1: Warm-Up: 3–5 mins cardio
DRILL 2: Mobility: 12-Exercise Sequence (2 x 30 secs each side)
DRILL 4: Cardio: Intervals (run/swim/row) 8 x 2 mins @ 90% max HR (3-min rest between intervals) • 3-min walk at end
DRILL 5: Cool Down: 6-Exercise Sequence (30 secs each)

WEDNESDAY

DRILL 1: Warm-Up: 3–5 mins cardio
DRILL 4: Cardio: Fuel Efficiency (run/swim/row) 50 mins @ 70% max HR • No food 8 hrs before or during session • 3-min walk at end
DRILL 5: Cool Down: 6-Exercise Sequence (30 secs each)

THURSDAY

DRILL 1: Warm-Up: 3–5 mins cardio
DRILL 2: Mobility: 12-Exercise Sequence (2 x 30 secs each side)
DRILL 3: Circuit Training: As Monday: 3 x (30 secs or 10 reps)
DRILL 5: Cool Down: 6-Exercise Sequence (30 secs each)

FRIDAY

DRILL 1: Warm-Up: 3–5 mins cardio
DRILL 2: Mobility: 12-Exercise Sequence (2 x 30 secs each side)
DRILL 1: Cardio: Intervals (run/swim/row) 5 x 5 mins @ 85% max HR (3-min rest between intervals) • 3-min walk at end
DRILL 5: Cool Down: 6-Exercise Sequence (30 secs each)

SATURDAY

DRILL 1: Warm-Up: 3–5 mins cardio
DRILL 2: Mobility: 12-Exercise Sequence (2 x 30 secs each side)
DRILL 4: Cardio: Recovery (run/swim/cycle) 30 mins @ 60% max HR
DRILL 5: Cool Down: 6-Exercise Sequence (30 secs each)

SUNDAY

DRILL 6: SMR: 14-Exercise Sequence (1 min each)

BERGEN TRAINING

In the P Company programme, one day of the week is focused on Bergen training. To prepare you for the conditions of P Company, the best training environment is mountainous terrain with uneven paths. When you feel ready, it should be very easy to create your own P Company-type events, which will give you great confidence. All you really need is a backpack and a suitable route. However, here are some tips to make the whole activity as safe and pain-free as possible.

Selecting a route

If you are going to venture into the hills, you will need to find a route that is both safe and the right distance. I would strongly recommend selecting a route which is predominantly made up of bridleways and is close to roads and civilization in case you get into trouble. A potential solution is completing laps of your local park, with a few hill reps thrown in for good measure. However, if you are attempting your own route somewhere off the beaten track here are some tips.

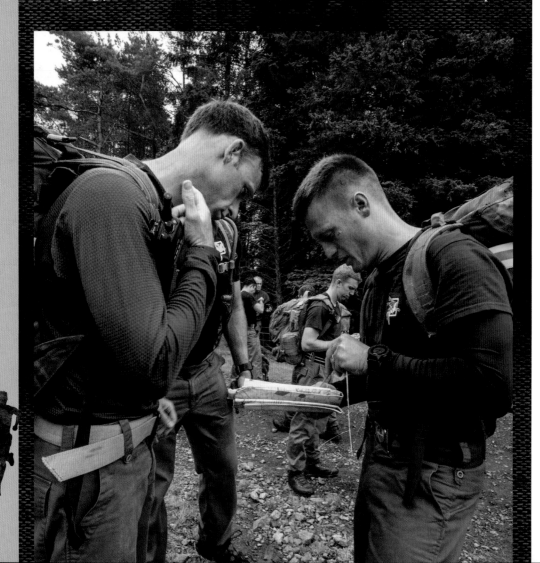

Navigation

For practical advice on how to map-read go on YouTube. Thereafter, it is important to have at least studied the route extensively before you set off, ideally using satellite imagery from Google Maps/Earth, which also gives you a sense of undulation. However, the best possible way to ensure you stay on track during a self-made P Company test is to recce it beforehand. Remember, time spent on recce is never wasted.

Kit requirements

Depending how off-track you venture, here are some items you might need:
- Bergen backpack, ideally with lumbar support and well-padded shoulder straps;
- first aid kit including plasters and zinc oxide tape;
- waterproof jacket and trousers;
- sleeping bag and waterproof bivvy bag;
- warm jumper/jacket or fleece;
- torch;
- hat and gloves;
- phone (for mountain rescue call 999 in the UK);
- food and water;
- spare socks;
- well worn-in walking boots (with ankle support);
- thick socks;
- CamelBak or equivalent water system;
- map (1:25,000 or 1:50,000);
- compass;
- GPS – optional and only in addition to a map and compass.

Bergen packing

When packing your Bergen your best bet is to have all your heavy stuff wrapped inside your sleeping bag, as this will reduce the risk of rubbing. After you have packed all essential equipment, weight is best made up with water, which is both useful and quick to dispose of safely if necessary.

Logistical support

When taking on a Bergen challenge, unless you are fortunate enough to have an appropriate testing ground, you will probably need to have some logistical support to make it work. The following is a list of resources which would significantly enhance the safety and enjoyment of your challenge:
- vehicle;
- driver with phone, map and knowledge of the route, and who knows what to do in the event of a problem;

- change of clothes;
- extra food and water for after the challenge.

Abort criteria

You should abort any Bergen march on remote areas in the event of the following:

- snow or ice (present or forecast);
- wind speed greater than 30mph;
- temperature either less than 1°C or greater than 20°C;
- driving rain;
- thick fog.

Injuries

If you are injured during the march, this is what you should do:

- Stop challenge and put on warm kit.
- Inform pre-determined safety person of your location (8-figure grid reference), type of injury, planned route off the hills, ETA.
- Treat injury if possible.
- Jettison any water being used for weight purposes, making sure you have sufficient drinking water.
- Make best possible speed to pre-agreed meeting point.
- Inform safety person when you are off the hills.
- Reattempt when appropriate.

Recreating test conditions

Unfortunately, sourcing a weapon will always be a problem and I wouldn't recommend it! An extra 10lb/4.5kg in your Bergen, which is considerably less annoying than carrying a long-barrelled weapon, is probably the best option.

P COMPANY TEST EVENTS: KEY INFORMATION

P Company Event/Distance	Height Lost/Gained	Time Allowed
2-miler	650ft	18 mins
10-miler	2,200ft	1 hr 50 mins
20-miler	4,300ft	4 hrs 10 mins

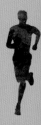
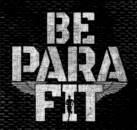

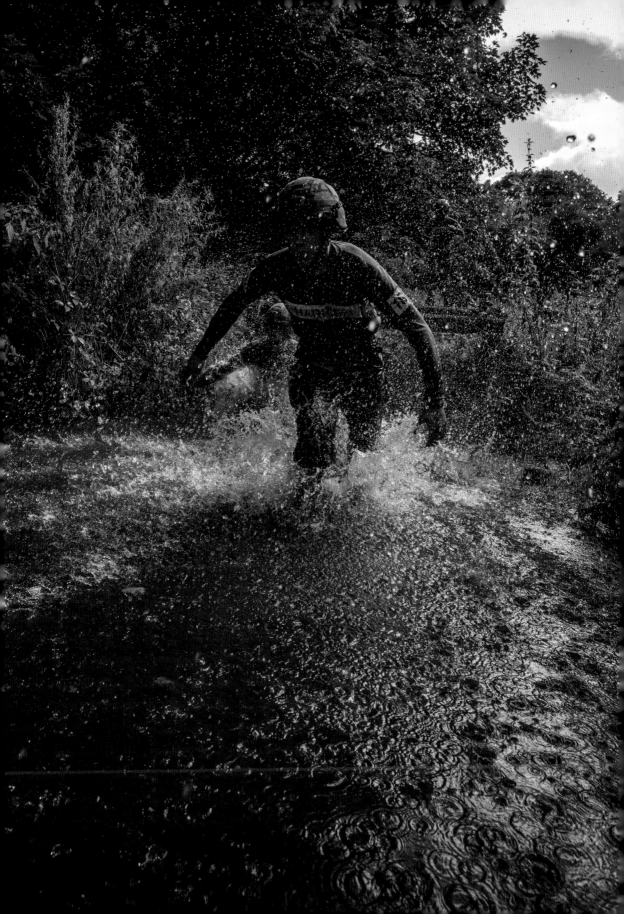

P COMPANY PROGRAMME

MONDAY

DRILL 1: **Warm-Up:** 3–5 mins cardio
DRILL 2: **Mobility:** 12-Exercise Sequence (2 x 30 secs each side)
Function Assessment: • As previous programmes
Cardio Assessment: (1 of 3) • Run or row 2.4km • Swim 750m
DRILL 3: **Circuit Training:** (max) • Pull-up • Standing jump • Press-up – 2 mins • Plank 3POC • Burpees – 1 min
DRILL 5: **Cool Down:** 6-Exercise Sequence (30 secs each)

TUESDAY

DRILL 6: **SMR:** 14-Exercise Sequence (1 min each)

WEDNESDAY

DRILL 1: **Warm-Up:** 3–5 mins cardio
DRILL 4: **Cardio:** Fuel Efficiency (run/swim/row) 50 mins @ 70% max HR • No food 8 hrs before or during session • 3-min walk at end
DRILL 5: **Cool Down:** 6-Exercise Sequence (30 secs each)

THURSDAY

DRILL 1: **Warm-Up:** 3–5 mins cardio
DRILL 2: **Mobility:** 12-Exercise Sequence (2 x 30 secs each side)
DRILL 3: **Circuit Training:** 3 x (30 secs or 10 reps) Superset • Twist (both sides)/vertical push • Horizontal pull/horizontal push • Vertical pull/squat • Bending pull/bending push • Plank (3POC)/burpees • Bear crawl
DRILL 5: **Cool Down:** 6-Exercise Sequence (30 secs each)

FRIDAY

DRILL 1: **Warm-Up:** 3–5 mins cardio
DRILL 2: **Mobility:** 12-Exercise Sequence (2 x 30 secs each side)
DRILL 4: **Cardio:** Bergen March (1st 4-week cycle) • 30 mins @ 70% max HR • 3-min walk at end • Bergen March (2nd 4-week cycle onwards) • 60 mins @ 70% max HR • 3-min walk at end
DRILL 5: **Cool Down**: 6-Exercise Sequence (30 secs each)

SATURDAY

DRILL 6: **SMR:** 14-Exercise Sequence (1 min each)

SUNDAY

DRILL 1: **Warm-Up:** 3–5 mins cardio
DRILL 2: **Mobility:** 12-Exercise Sequence (2 x 30 secs each side)
DRILL 4: **Cardio:** Intervals (run/swim/cycle) 5 x 5 mins @ 90% max HR (3-min rest between intervals) • 3-min walk at end
DRILL 5: **Cool Down:** 6-Exercise Sequence (30 secs each)

WEEK 2 (LOAD)

MONDAY

DRILL 1: Warm-Up: 3–5 mins cardio
DRILL 2: Mobility: 12-Exercise Sequence (2 x 30 secs each side)
DRILL 3: Circuit Training: 3 x (30 secs or 10 reps) Superset • Twist (both sides)/vertical push • Horizontal pull/horizontal push • Vertical pull/squat • Bending pull/bending push • Plank (3POC)/burpees • Bear crawl
DRILL 5: Cool Down: 6-Exercise Sequence (30 secs each)

TUESDAY

DRILL 1: Warm-Up: 3–5 mins cardio
DRILL 2: Mobility: 12-Exercise Sequence (2 x 30 secs each side)
DRILL 4: Cardio: Intervals (run /swim/row) 8 x 2 mins @ 90% max HR (3-min rest between intervals) • 3-min walk at end
DRILL 5: Cool Down: 6-Exercise Sequence (30 secs each)

WEDNESDAY

DRILL 1: Warm-Up: 3–5 mins cardio
DRILL 4: Cardio: Fuel Efficiency (run/swim/row) 50 mins @ 70% max HR • No food 8 hrs before or during session • 3-min walk at end
DRILL 5: Cool Down: 6-Exercise Sequence (30 secs each)

THURSDAY

DRILL 1: Warm-Up: 3–5 mins cardio
DRILL 2: Mobility: 12-Exercise Sequence (2 x 30 secs each side)
DRILL 3: Circuit Training: As Monday: 3 x (30 secs or 10 reps)
DRILL 5: Cool Down: 6-Exercise Sequence (30 secs each)

FRIDAY

DRILL 1: Warm-Up: 3–5 mins cardio
DRILL 4: Cardio: Bergen March (1st 4-week cycle) • 60 mins @ 70% max HR • 3-min walk at end • Bergen March (2nd 4-week cycle onwards) • 120 mins @ 70% max HR • 3-min walk at end
DRILL 5: Cool Down: 6-Exercise Sequence (30 secs each)

SATURDAY

DRILL 6: SMR: 14-Exercise Sequence (1 min each)

SUNDAY

DRILL 1: Warm-Up: 3–5 mins cardio
DRILL 2: Mobility: 12-Exercise Sequence (2 x 30 secs each side)
DRILL 4: Cardio: Intervals (run/swim/cycle) 5 x 5 mins @ 90% max HR (3-min rest between intervals) • 3-min walk at end
DRILL 5: Cool Down: 6-Exercise Sequence (30 secs each)

P COMPANY PROGRAMME

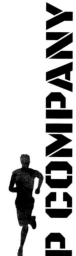

MONDAY

DRILL 1: Warm-Up: 3–5 mins cardio
DRILL 2: Mobility: 12-Exercise Sequence (2 x 30 secs each side)
DRILL 3: Circuit Training: 3 x (30 secs or 10 reps) Superset • Twist (both sides)/vertical push • Horizontal pull/horizontal push • Vertical pull/squat • Bending pull/bending push • Plank (3POC)/burpees • Bear crawl
DRILL 5: Cool Down: 6-Exercise Sequence (30 secs each)

TUESDAY

DRILL 1: Warm-Up: 3–5 mins cardio
DRILL 2: Mobility: 12-Exercise Sequence (2 x 30 secs each side)
DRILL 4: Cardio: Intervals (run /swim/row) 8 x 2 mins @ 90% max HR (3-min rest between intervals) • 3-min walk at end
DRILL 5: Cool Down: 6-Exercise Sequence (30 secs each)

WEDNESDAY

DRILL 1: Warm-Up: 3–5 mins cardio
DRILL 4: Cardio: Fuel Efficiency (run/swim/row) 50 mins @ 70% max HR • No food 8 hrs before or during session • 3-min walk at end
DRILL 5: Cool Down: 6-Exercise Sequence (30 secs each)

THURSDAY

DRILL 1: Warm-Up: 3–5 mins cardio
DRILL 2: Mobility: 12-Exercise Sequence (2 x 30 secs each side)
DRILL 3: Circuit Training: As Monday: 3 x (30 secs or 10 reps)
DRILL 5: Cool Down: 6-Exercise Sequence (30 secs each)

FRIDAY

DRILL 1: Warm-Up: 3–5 mins cardio
DRILL 4: Cardio: Bergen March (1st 4-week cycle) • 90 mins @ 70% max HR • 3-min walk at end • Bergen March (2nd 4-week cycle onwards) • 120 mins @ 70% max HR • 3-min walk at end
DRILL 5: Cool Down: 6-Exercise Sequence (30 secs each)

SATURDAY

DRILL 6: SMR: 14-Exercise Sequence (1 min each)

SUNDAY

DRILL 1: Warm-Up: 3–5 mins cardio
DRILL 2: Mobility: 12-Exercise Sequence (2 x 30 secs each side)
DRILL 4: Cardio: Intervals (run/swim/cycle) 5 x 5 mins @ 90% max HR (3-min rest between intervals) • 3-min walk at end
DRILL 5: Cool Down: 6-Exercise Sequence (30 secs each)

WEEK 4 (DE-LOAD)

MONDAY

DRILL 1: Warm-Up: 3–5 mins cardio
DRILL 2: Mobility: 12-Exercise Sequence (2 x 30 secs each side)
DRILL 3: Circuit Training: 3 x (30 secs or 10 reps) Superset • Twist (both sides)/vertical push • Horizontal pull/horizontal push • Vertical pull/squat • Bending pull/bending push • Plank (3POC)/burpees • Bear crawl
DRILL 5: Cool Down: 6-Exercise Sequence (30 secs each)

TUESDAY

DRILL 1: Warm-Up: 3–5 mins cardio
DRILL 2: Mobility: 12-Exercise Sequence (2 x 30 secs each side)
DRILL 4: Cardio: Intervals (run /swim/row) 8 x 2 mins @ 90% max HR (3-min rest between intervals) • 3-min walk at end
DRILL 5: Cool Down: 6-Exercise Sequence (30 secs each)

WEDNESDAY

DRILL 1: Warm-Up: 3–5 mins cardio
DRILL 2: Mobility: 12-Exercise Sequence (2 x 30 secs each side)
DRILL 4: Cardio: Recovery (run/swim/cycle) 30 mins @ 60% max HR
DRILL 5: Cool Down: 6-Exercise Sequence (30 secs each)

THURSDAY

DRILL 1: Warm-Up: 3–5 mins cardio
DRILL 2: Mobility: 12-Exercise Sequence (2 x 30 secs each side)
DRILL 3: Circuit Training: As Monday: 3 x (30 secs or 10 reps)
DRILL 5: Cool Down: 6-Exercise Sequence (30 secs each)

FRIDAY

DRILL 1: Warm-Up: 3–5 mins cardio
DRILL 4: Cardio: Bergen March (1st 4-week cycle) • 60 mins @ 70% max HR • 3-min walk at end • Bergen March (2nd 4-week cycle onwards) • 90 mins @ 70% max HR • 3-min walk at end
DRILL 5: Cool Down: 6-Exercise Sequence (30 secs each)

SATURDAY

DRILL 6: SMR: 14-Exercise Sequence (1 min each)

SUNDAY

DRILL 1: Warm-Up: 3–5 mins cardio
DRILL 2: Mobility: 12-Exercise Sequence (2 x 30 secs each side)
DRILL 4: Cardio: Recovery (run/swim/cycle) 30 mins @ 60% max HR
DRILL 5: Cool Down: 6-Exercise Sequence (30 secs each)

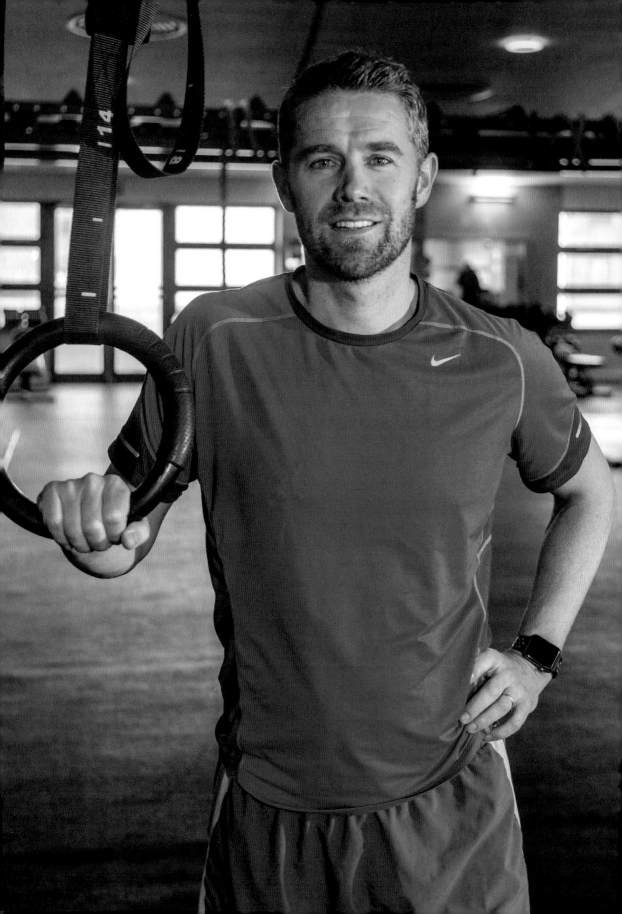

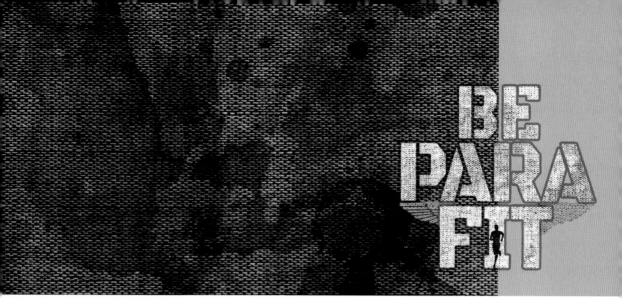

Chapter 5

FORCE MULTIPLIERS:
FITNESS AIDS

In this section I want to provide some guidance on other resources you can access to support you in scaling my fitness programmes or with your own specific stretch goal. But first a word of caution. How you transform your physical fitness is a complex question, which all too often people replace with a simpler question, such as: where can I get fit or who can help me get fit? **Thinking fast vs slow is the error that enables many gyms to sell memberships and personal trainer packages that go unused.** Be warned – they're impotent in isolation. Nothing in this chapter is a substitute for the pyramid approach described over the last four chapters – fitness is a system which requires a systematic approach. What follows are merely some resources that can help you, but only after you have secured solid foundations of sleep, nutrition and mobility, and have progressed to Level 2: Fighting Fit.

GYMS

The right gym has the potential to be the ideal venue to hone fitness and make friends with a ready-made support network. But before you even set foot in one, you must first define what you need from a gym, so you can select it on that basis and maximize its value. Once you are clear what you need from a gym, I would urge you to consider ease of use, cost and service when selecting the right one.

EASE OF USE

It is essential that your gym fits around your lifestyle. Being located close to work, home, or at least en route is a critical success factor. Make sure you go to the gym knowing exactly what you want from it and when you intend to use it, and don't be seduced by the honey trap of a good-looking sales person playing to your ego. Look for potential pitfalls – if you're struggling to make it fit, then even the smallest friction will stop you using it. Before you sign-up, do a full dress rehearsal of a gym session at exactly the time you intend to train in order to assess the following:

- location – transit time, parking and access;
- opening hours – early morning is essential for pre-work sessions;
- occupancy during your intended training windows – availability of lockers/time spent waiting for equipment, etc.

SERVICE

Gyms provide a service and it is important to find one that supports your goals and is configured for your convenience. An ancient military maxim is 'time spent on reconnaissance is never wasted'; this is equally true when scoping out gyms. During your recce, look out for the following:

- How is the gym organized? Is it efficient and well run?
- What equipment does it have? What state is it in and how does it compare with what you're looking for?
- Do the staff and other members make you feel comfortable?
- What do the other members say about the staff?
- What qualifications do the staff have and what classes do they offer?
- A good test is asking what happens if you forget your membership card – if their answer is a penalty fee or they deny you access, take your business elsewhere.

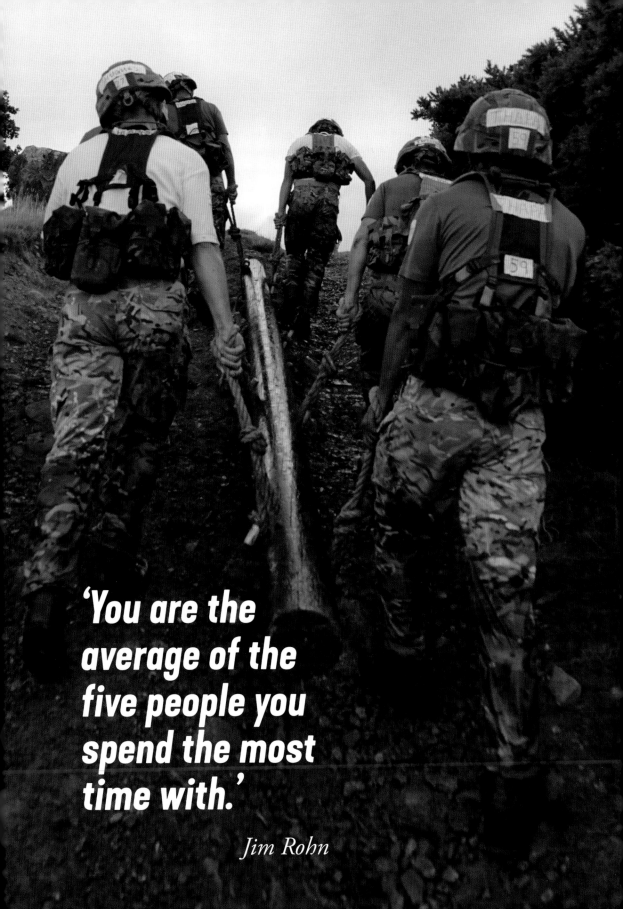

'You are the average of the five people you spend the most time with.'

Jim Rohn

COST

Gym memberships are priced to attract people to join for an extended period (normally a year) because statistically most clients won't use the gym much after mid-January. If all you want is weights, a locker and a shower, then all additional services are a waste of your membership fees. You will pay a premium for prime-time usage, but if you were planning to only use the gym at off-peak times, you may be able to purchase a cheaper membership that includes the relevant time window. My personal requirements from a gym are:

- provides towel and shower gel;
- access to permanent locker to store your office clothes and toiletries, essential for run/cycle commuting;
- training attire, which significantly reduces washing bill and need to carry soiled clothing between home and office. I run home in the gym attire, then run in wearing it the following day;
- limited waiting time for equipment.

PERSONAL TRAINERS

If you can afford a personal trainer, a good one can significantly enhance the effectiveness of your exercise programme. All reputable gyms' personal trainers will have relevant local qualifications, which ensures a level of training literacy & coaching proficiency. Personal trainers should be used to provide expertise on technical form, drive you to invest in mobility as part of your training and provide best practice advice based on their closeness to advances in training methodologies. Using a personal trainer for companionship or to just get you to the gym will be an expensive folly, unlikely to drive significant improvements in your training. You are looking for someone to blend authentic support with challenge in order to aid your development – anything else doesn't warrant either the financial investment or the effort of synchronizing your schedule with theirs for the session.

CREDIBILITY

Your relationship with your personal trainer is a critical success factor. Mutual trust, confidentiality, empathy and acceptance of your goals and ability are all key. Equally important is your personal trainer's credibility and confidence (but not ego), which will enhance your confidence in them. For me, the most important factor is role modelling. Your personal trainer needs to practice what they preach and have the experience of having trained hard for a specific goal over an extended period – otherwise how else can they understand what you will be going through? Pay for a trial session, to assess their suitability. I would suggest the following questions:

- What are they training for; do they put their own theory into practice?
- What are their specialties? If your focus is aerobic endurance, then a powerlifter will have little to offer.
- What personal development training have they done in the last three months, and what are they doing in the next three months?
- What are the last three training books they read?
- What is their time management like; when is the last time they overslept or had a session run more than 5 minutes over time?

Once you have found one you like, ask for a coffee to discuss your training objectives for the next three months and ask them to codify the training programme they will design for the first month during your first session.

If a personal trainer ever does any of the following during a session, look for another: checks social media on their phone; puts you on treadmill except to test fitness; is unable to articulate what a session's objectives are as part of the broader training plan.

I had a personal trainer for about three years to help me improve my mobility and strength and complement my ultra-running. At the height of our work together we met three times per week before work. I selected Isaac having observed his professionalism with his other clients. I interviewed him over a green juice, liked him and saw his value instantly. From the outset he significantly improved the quality of my gym sessions, and brought me up-to-date on training theory and practice. However, as we started at 6am, the only slot he had available, I was up at 5am to make the appointment and found myself often compromising my sleep to make the session. Over time, as demand for his services grew and my running volume increased, synchronizing our schedules became difficult. I also felt that I'd embedded his session repertoire and was able to achieve 90% of what we'd do together on my own. So in the end I decided to buy gym equipment and train at home. This not only saved me time as well as money in the medium term, but it enabled me to have breakfast with my daughters between training and going to work on strength days, which I enjoy all the more.

Both gyms and personal trainers are expensive luxuries and should be treated as such. Moreover, if something designed to improve your health puts you under time and financial stress, you're prescribing a fatal cure. Look for a solution that fits your financial means and available time and avoids any long-term financial commitment. A great course of action might be to use a personal trainer to help you refine your own home routine and master the core functional movement patterns, to prevent the risk of injury. In just 1–2 sessions a good personal trainer will help you construct a programme tailored to your fitness level, available time and that doesn't require access to a gym. In the remainder of the chapter I'll cover three more options that have the potential to transform your fitness level without breaking the bank:

- sports clubs/teams;
- fitness technology;
- virtual/online coaches.

SPORT CLUBS/TEAMS

While having your own personal trainer sounds impressive, significant research favours being part of a team. When it comes to embedding training into your life and bridging the gap between novice and advanced elite athlete, clubs win nine times out of ten. Whether running, cycling, triathlon, Boot Camp, CrossFit or anything else with a competitive edge, joining a good club/team is your best means of improving your performance. The main benefits are:

- **Accountability.** Being part of a team/community creates both accountability and a support network. You're more likely to keep going when others are counting on you and will support you to achieve your goals.
- **Consistency.** The steady cadence of weekly or even daily sessions normalizes training as a habit and fosters commitment.
- **Structured training.** Teams/clubs often provide access to specialized training such as coached technical sessions or facilitated interval sessions. Use a club to support you on the more difficult aspects of your training programme so you can tackle the easier training on your own. Your discipline is in turning up, not devising the plan for the session.
- **Motivation.** Having a frequent dose of competition between races spurs you to train harder. Chasing someone faster/stronger than you or knowing someone is hot on your heels causes you to push yourself harder than you would on your own. Subconsciously, a phenomenon described as 'social facilitation' happens – in other words, training in a group results in you becoming consumed by the activity, recognizing neither the effort nor pain as much as you would do on your own.
- **Learning environment.** The collective wisdom of a group of people committed to achieving similar goals has multiple benefits. Teams help provide signposts to competitions, new training methodologies and training routes as well as critical feedback on new equipment and technologies. Together you all learn from each other's success and failures.

Like every training aid, understanding the club/team's part in your training programme is essential. For instance, if training is a source of solitude and introspection a club will be counterproductive. The main challenge with any club, beyond its quality, is synchronizing your schedule to accommodate it into your own battle rhythm. Once you have determined that joining a club is right for you, I would advocate a full dress rehearsal using the criteria defined within the gym section to assess whether a specific club is right for you.

Despite being a strong advocate of training clubs, I don't currently use them myself. The age of my children means they are in bed around 7.30pm, the time most clubs would be in full throttle. While getting out of work on time is not an issue, seeing my kids before bedtime is. By saying 'yes' to the club, I'm saying 'no' to them. In isolation this would be fine one night a week, but my job requires at least two mid-week evening commitments that mean I don't see my girls before bed. I also do quite a bit of mid-week business travel. So, for the time being clubs aren't for me, but I plan to integrate one when my kids are older. In other words, both how you train and where you train should fit your current circumstances and evolve with life.

FITNESS TECHNOLOGY
FITNESS APPS

Technology is revolutionizing the fitness industry at an accelerated rate, by providing cheap access to the most advanced training systems and processes. Smartphones have been transformational in providing access to training content, tracking activity, and connecting people with each other, coaches and elite athletes. Your phone is instantly capable of helping you significantly improve your fitness and general health at little or no cost.

Activity and nutrition trackers

The base of the pyramid is founded on sleep, nutrition and mobility habits. These are all perfectly addressed by using wearable technology such as Fitbits, smart watches and phones. All provide efficient means to track and optimize your patterns of behaviour to support a healthier lifestyle. These apps are increasingly interconnected, with one dashboard providing access to your sleep, nutrition, standing habits, training activity and calorie consumption data. Apps such as myfitnesspal routinely include the nutritional content of all food types and quantities, including the menus of most restaurant chains. Tracking your health data has never been cheaper or easier: you get what you measure.

I personally use an Apple phone and the Apple health app to track my movement. A few years ago I tracked my nutrition for about two months using myfitnesspal to develop a better understanding of how well my diet serviced my macro nutritional requirements. Two months gave me sufficient time to cover the full spectrum of my diet and track how it changed during business travel and family holidays. The process of logging my food and how I felt afterwards also helped me develop an understanding of how different foods make me feel. At first the process took me 2–3 minutes per meal, but quickly became less than a minute as the app stored all my previous meals and was well worth the time investment. After reviewing my personal results, I increased my consumption of vegetables and significantly reduced my intake of milk and processed bread and continue to feel much better for it.

Training content applications

Training applications are the modern equivalent of the DVD home fitness collection, but accessible anywhere anytime from your smartphone. From cross-fit to yoga, all tastes are catered for, with coaches uploading free content online via YouTube or Facebook as well as more traditional downloadable apps. There are a countless number of free and subscription-based apps offering an array of services, which amount to cheap, easy access to training programmes and exercise instructions. Nike Training Club and Vitogo are examples of apps that provide access to an exhaustive database of programmes, exercise instructions and motivation. The key considerations for these apps are as follows:

Strengths
- Provide access to content, cheaply and conveniently.
- Have built-in ability to track training activity.
- Help with motivation by streaming content from inspiring role models and training experts.

Weaknesses
- Lack of regulation results in varying quality and many unfounded claims on their effectiveness. We instinctively want to believe a fitness application is the solution to all our fitness goals, but there is no substitute for discipline in following a fitness- and nutrition-based programme. Like a personal coach, paying a premium should provide no reassurance of effectiveness.
- As detailed earlier, the training process relies on each session having an objective and being aligned to an overarching performance goal.

All sessions should be mutually supporting, with progress earnt from every constituent session. This means fitness apps work best when the user is training literate and using it to address a specific training objective as part of a structured programme. Alternatively, activity should be project managed by a coach with the necessary expertise to select and combine activities effectively to reduce risk of injury or time wasted on junk activities that serve no broader purpose.

- There could be data privacy issues from apps that allow unrestricted access to your activity and phone content. Be warned if you're not paying for the app: you are the product and their business model is selling your data to any bidder no matter what their motive.

On the basis that you're far more likely to take a phone than a book to the gym, I have sought to incorporate all of the strengths from apps and activity trackers identified above into the design of the Be PARA Fit app to maximize your training effectiveness. My app provides a bespoke training programme tailored to your specific fitness level and allows you to integrate it with other health apps, so you're able to track your training alongside monitoring your sleep, nutrition and movement.

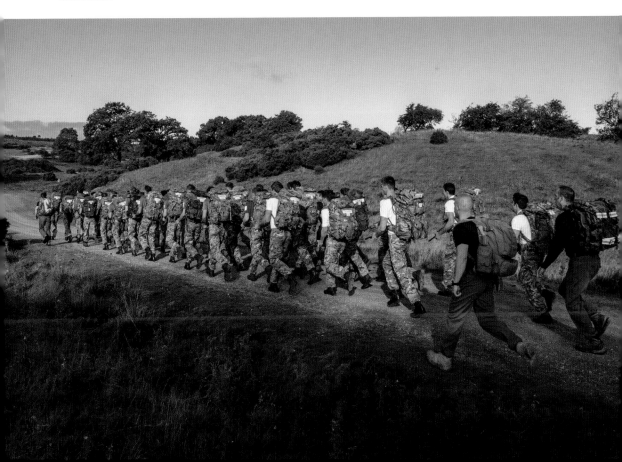

Virtual training applications and communities

A distinct branch of fitness apps that warrants special mention are virtual tracking training applications. Examples include Strava, Nike Training Club and Fitbit. These apps enable athletes and coaches to engage within a broader training community and are the best proxy for being a part of a training group, when geography or schedules prevent training with others. Gone are the days of requiring a cumbersome GPS watch to capture a trail run. All apps can now be downloaded to a smartphone or watch, with all activity instantly uploaded subject to being connected to the Internet.

Key considerations:

- Opportunity to undertake individualized workouts, which fit with your schedule.
- Work best when integrated into a structured training programme.
- Opportunity to share goals, offer support, compete and track progress with friends, without the need to synchronize activity.
- Cheap and easy means of logging all activity and tracking progress across multiple metrics (distance, speed, time, HR, calories, watt output).
- Summarizes progress and activities (training volume, personal bests, course records).
- Facilitates connectivity with virtual coach.
- Access to subscription to free challenges (e.g. run a set distance in a week).
- Safety beacon options enable others to track you while running, so they can estimate your return or come to you in an emergency.
- Opportunity to follow elite athletes' activity and search for interesting training routes.
- Premium membership offers increased analytics and access to advanced training content.

I use Strava extensively to track my running and Wattbike cycling. I really like all the analytics available on the Strava Premium version and find it helps me improve my training. While I don't actively chase course records on Strava, I confess to being annoyed whenever I lose one!

VIRTUAL/ONLINE COACHES

Virtual coaches provide the ability to outsource the technical thought of building a training programme to achieve a specific training objective at a vastly reduced price. The combination of web-based training software and virtual training communities enables athletes to transcend differences in distance and even time zones to engage with world-class experts. Coaches are able to provide dynamic weekly training programmes, by monitoring training activity and performance online.

Key considerations:

- Ideal when life commitments or your location preclude joining and training with a club or team.
- Work best in a competitive sport like running, cycling, swimming, or rowing where training activity can be shared using online technologies.
- Virtual coaches are considerably less effective in gym-based training, where providing guidance on form is key and capturing training activity is more difficult from technology.
- Suitable if you are at an intermediate level, literate in the sport with decent form, and you are able to motivate yourself to train on your own.
- Most elite athletes, save the top few, supplement their income as virtual coaches. This gives you the added benefit of feeling you are supporting an elite athlete with your own training.
- The sweet spot is someone ranked 50–100 globally in their sport, who speaks the same language and is ideally in the same time zone. You want someone who is dedicated to their sport but relies on their coaching as an income source, making them more reliable.
- Most have an online presence and their own training website, so you can connect with them.
- Like selecting a personal trainer, know what you want from them and avoid being seduced by a great athlete who is a poor coach. Request a Skype/Facetime conversation for you both to decide if there is a mutual fit. I would recommend using the criteria defined within the personal trainer section to help you.

I have used an online coach for nearly three years. My coach Vlad Ixel is currently ranked first in his age group for 70.3 triathlon and 25th globally for trail ultra-marathons. I benefit from having access to a great coach and the knowledge that a world-class athlete is helping me achieve my training objectives. Meanwhile, Vlad is able to supplement his income en route to achieving his own, considerably more aggressive, training objectives. Our relationship has had a profound impact on my training and performance. When the time is right, I'd strongly recommend replicating this with a virtual coach of your own.

TRAINING IN COMBAT ZONES AND CORPORATE LIFE

I've used the full spectrum of fitness facilities over my six operational deployments as a paratrooper, but Afghanistan stands out. In the immediate aftermath of the terrorist attacks on the Twin Towers in 2001, I was among the first soldiers to enter Kabul. My platoon – 10 Platoon, D Company, 2 PARA – was a hardy band of men, with a mutual respect and trust fused by demanding training and common purpose. On deployment, we were the holders of the Bruneval Cup, a competition fiercely fought out to identify 2 PARA's best platoon. We'd won the title largely down to our fitness, which was exceptional even by Parachute Regiment standards. This fitness had been hard to attain and we were all equally committed to preserving it during our emergency deployment to Afghanistan.

Maintenance of morale

From our quarters in a bombed-out former Russian barracks in Kabul, I observed the sort of ingenuity and resourcefulness that is the trademark of airborne soldiers. Using a selection of equipment that was either bought from the local bazaar, or borrowed and misused from the quartermaster's department, we created a gym within a week of arriving. In the months that followed, our improvised gym not only kept us fit for our demanding patrol programme but provided some escapism from the intense Taliban insurgency we were fighting against. The hours we spent in our makeshift gym were social occasions and a daily ritual. Looking back, it was as much about relieving the stress of the day through aggressive banter as it was about coming together to beat yesterday's performance and push one another.

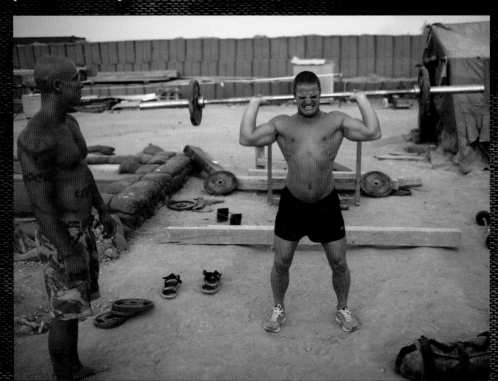

Several years later, when deployed a few hours down the road in Helmand Province, I noticed that along with the rest of the infrastructure, military gyms had come on a long way; the norm was now aircraft hangars filled with state-of-the-art fitness equipment. But their purpose was the same – keeping soldiers mentally and physically fit to fight tomorrow's challenges.

Enduring operations

While my days may no longer be punctuated by tactical planning briefs and counter-insurgency operations, the daily ritual of pushing myself physically remains a constant. I prioritize training like any important meeting and protect it at all costs. It's an approach that many of my corporate colleagues struggle with, and one I always address the same way. If my people and clients want me at my best, then a daily dose of training is as important as me having slept the night before.

Training provides order to my day, offers respite and gives me perspective from work matters. It is a source of inspiration that nourishes all parts of my life. I train to connect with people – those united by a philosophy of self-improvement, not a postcode. Being around people with a younger mindset (physically and intellectually) not only drives me physically to perform better but creates unique insights both personally and professionally.

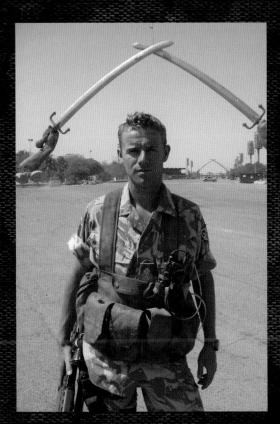

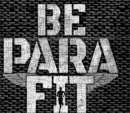

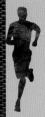

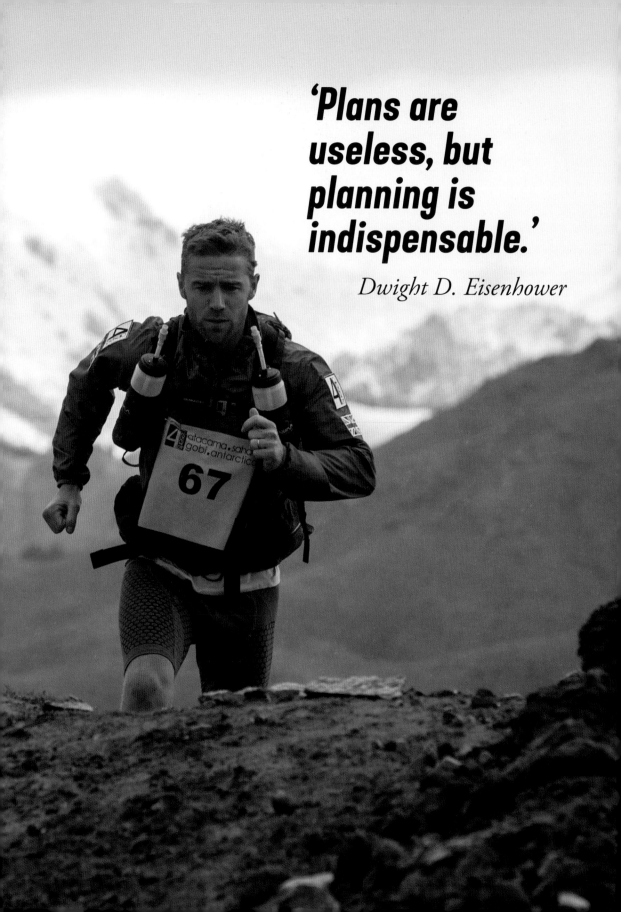

'**Plans are useless, but planning is indispensable.**'

Dwight D. Eisenhower

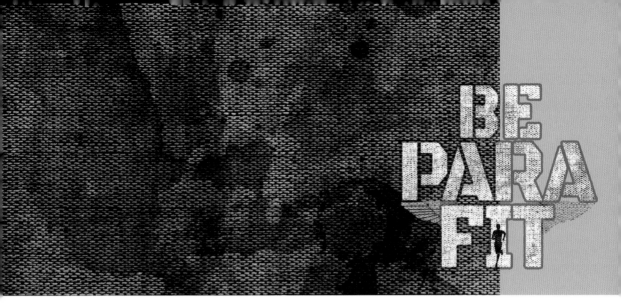

CHAPTER 6

FIT FOR LIFE:
EFFECTIVE GOAL-SETTING

INTEGRATING FITNESS INTO A BUSY LIFE

Every January I'm filled with hope when I hear friends committing to ambitious goals to turn the tide in the year ahead – to make more time for family and fitness and spend less time in the office. Sadly, most lose momentum by February, by simply repeating last year's mistakes – confusing *how* to get fit with *where* to get fit and buying an expensive gym membership that's rarely used. **Any fitness programme, trainer or gym equipment will be impotent without sufficient training time and a lifestyle that supports it**. The focus of this chapter is not your specific training goal but a framework to help you appropriately prioritize training so it fits your personal circumstances, and then find space for it.

The approach I describe is one I have developed and fine-tuned since leaving the PARAs to keep me fighting fit and comfortably in the top ten of all of the ultra-marathons I compete in. But first a caveat – I don't believe in balance; it's a mythical prize that creates incredible stress and self-judgement in all who pursue it. It's impossible to be all things, to all people, all of the time – different goals demand a different level of focus on different days. My aim is to be present: fully immersed in whatever I'm doing, wherever I am, whomever I'm with. And as for balance, the steeper your learning curve and the further you reach, the more it will be disturbed.

THE TRANSITION FROM PARATROOPER TO CORPORATE WARRIOR

A decade ago fitness was an integral part of my profession, my life was simple, and I had an abundance of time to devote to training. Fast forward to the present and things couldn't be more different, not that I'd change it. Undoubtedly there are similarities between my past military life and my current civilian life, not least a performance culture that drives high-calibre people to link arms and achieve

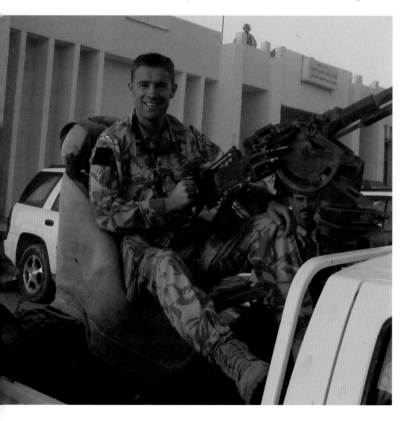
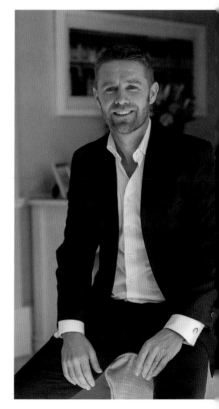

audacious goals. However, an early insight was that unlike the PARAs, neither my new peers nor the companies they worked for connected sleeping well, eating well or training with commercial success. Within a year I found the rhythm of corporate life corrosive to my health: 11–13 hours at a desk, wedded to a smartphone, late-night conference calls, client entertainment, long-haul travel, to say nothing of the numerous family milestones missed or not enjoyed due to a preoccupation with work. Facing an early crossroads in my new career, I decided I wasn't prepared to sacrifice my health for wealth. I took a day to think and plan how best to integrate a demanding physical regime into my new life, then set about implementing it; a week later every aspect of my life was richer for it.

To find time to master fitness, you need to understand its relative importance against countless other priorities. I believe your success, like mine, will be built on deploying focus and order to your life, so **training complements rather than competes with your work and family commitments**. There is no instant formula for greatness. Grappling with difficult questions is the price you must pay for success: how hard are you prepared to work for it and what are you willing to sacrifice to achieve it? We'll be striving for hundreds of marginal gains – progress, not necessarily perfection. The fundamentals of our approach will draw on two key concepts, both products of a military recipe for success that's been perfected over generations: mission analysis and optimizing your battle rhythm.

MISSION ANALYSIS

Mission analysis is the launchpad for all military objectives – a process focused on precisely defining and refining our mission, building the best plan to achieve it, and then weighing what we expect to win against what we risk. In the PARAs we use war-gaming, a type of pre-mortem, to pick apart our planning process, which spurs creativity, innovation and ultimately a better plan. We then use rehearsals to help us develop a practical understanding of potential weaknesses in the plan, so we can optimize it further before it's exposed to the enemy. Mission analysis helps us determine:

1. The **critical steps** necessary to achieve the objective.
2. The **resources** (time, equipment, money, support etc) required to accomplish each mission essential task – in particular, how to maximize the available resources.
3. **When** and **where** activities need to take place in relation to one another to maximize the chance of success.
4. **Mission viability** – is the expected prize worth the price?

GOALS SYNC MATRIX

	Fitness	Career	Personal
Ideal			
Now			
3–5-Year Goals			
1-Year Goals			
Time			
Money			
Minimum Standard			

KEY

Ideal: Define what what constitutes 10 out of 10 for each goal.
Now: Rate yourself now out of 10 against your ideal state.
3–5-Year Goals: Identify 1–3 things that take you closer to your ideal state.
1-Year Goals: Define 1–3 things that get you closer to your 3–5 year goals.
Time: Capture weekly time associated with your 1-year goals.
Money: Assess costs associated with your 1-year goals.
Minimum Standard: Define minimum standards you will hold yourself to in all circumstances.

MANAGING MULTIPLE GOALS

In the PARAs we typically have multiple missions running concurrently in the battle space. In order to manage our resources effectively we use a sync matrix to help us visualize and understand all our moving parts. In a similar vein, every personal goal we pursue must struggle for time and attention amid our other commitments. A sync matrix like the above example helps me understand how all of my goals in various aspects of life interact and potentially compete with one another.

SCHEDULING

The next step for me after the sync matric is scheduling, which in practice is a highly interdependent exercise. I find it's really only when I plot and track all of my goals on an annual planner that I'm able to determine what's possible and edit appropriately. Once I've given this a first pass, my wife and I sit down and fine-tune it to ensure it is adapted for the good of the family. Last year was a great year for us – I attribute much of this to taking time to define and refine our goals together. I highly recommend performing this exercise to capture, schedule and agree all the things you are committed to achieving with those closest to you.

APPLICATION TO TRAINING

Any enduring training goal requires a permanent change for it to be successful. While difficult, change is made easier when you're able to anticipate the various obstacles and challenges you will face and rally all available resources to maximize your chances of success. The logic underlying the mission analysis process is designed to find the best solution for executing complex, multi-phase tasks with limited resources. **Whether fighting a fierce enemy or a sedentary lifestyle, applying time and rigour to understand your adversary and maximize your available resources is the surest route to victory.** All four mission analysis criteria and the thinking they stimulate are directly applicable to weighing fitness goals against the competing demands of a busy life. To bring the mission analysis process to life in a fitness context, I have included an example of my current training goal on pages 174–175 to help guide and inspire you to apply a similar approach to planning the success of your own goals.

FITNESS STANDARDS AND LIFESTYLE CHOICES

The table on the following page is designed to help you understand the lifestyle considerations of different levels of fitness, so you can work out what is right for you now. As I have said before and you'll note in the table, fitness follows a diminishing returns profile; the fitter you get, the harder you have to work and the more you have to sacrifice to gain each increment of fitness. Be true to yourself and those around you when picking your target. As the book title suggests, I believe the sweet spot is Paratrooper Fitness.

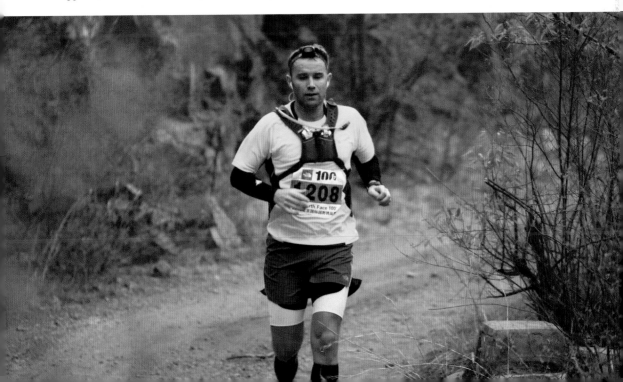

PHYSIQUE

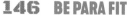

FITNESS STANDARD: **Sedentary <50th percentile**
Sleep: No sleep consistency
Nutrition: Little/no nutritional planning • Diet high in refined carbohydrates, deep-fried foods, alcohol • Large portions • Eat quickly • No fasting except when sleeping
Mobility: Limited daily movement • No stretching • **Consequence**: Poor posture and weak core • Lower-back issues • Restricted range of motion in joints • Prone to injury without exertion
Training: Little/no training activity
Mindset: Health and appearance may impact self-confidence • Unable to enjoy any exertion
Mission Analysis: No dedicated time and effort to maintain, but hidden costs are severe: Activity leaves breathless • Poor health & low life expectancy • Prone to depression

FITNESS STANDARD: **Active >50–75th percentile**
Sleep: 7 hrs most nights
Nutrition: Nutrition planned/achieved 70% of the time • Restrict alcohol/processed foods to 2 portions per day • Eat slowly some of the time • 3L of water per day • Eat within 14-hr window
Mobility: Infrequent movement during the day • 15 mins stretching 2–3 x per week •
Consequence: Posture impacted by prolonged sitting and lazy core muscles • Good range of motion in major joints • Prone to injure in intense activity or abnormal movement patterns
Training: 2–3 x 30-min+ sessions 3 x per week with no hard sessions
Mindset: Feel healthy and energetic most of the time • Enjoy activity • Confident in appearance
Mission Analysis: Requires small investments in training time, effort and lifestyle choices for significant improvements in health and lifespan • Easy to maintain at any stage of life

FITNESS STANDARD: **Fit >75–95th percentile**
Sleep: 7 hrs every night
Nutrition: Nutrition planned/achieved 80% of the time • Restrict alcohol/processed foods to 1 portion per day • Eat slowly most of the time • 3L of water per day • Eat within 12-hr window
Mobility: Move throughout the day • 15 mins stretching (inc SMR) 5 x per week • **Consequence:** Good posture • Good range of motion in all joints • May injure in intense activity or abnormal movement patterns
Training: 5 x 30-min+ sessions per week including 1–2 hard sessions
Mindset: Feel strong and energetic • Sense of purpose and pride in appearance • Enjoy being associated with fitness • Grit developed from hard sessions boosts confidence in other areas of life
Mission Analysis: Requires small but frequent investments in training time, effort and lifestyle choices • Optimal health range • Improves mental resilience • Easy to maintain at any stage of life

FITNESS STANDARD: **Paratrooper >95 percentile**
Sleep: 8 hrs most nights
Nutrition: Nutrition planned/achieved 90% of time • Restrict processed food/alcohol to 5 portions per week • Eat slowly all of the time • 4L of water daily • Eat within 11-hr window
Mobility: Move throughout the day • 15 mins stretching (inc SMR) 5 x per week • **Consequence:** Excellent posture • Full range of motion in all joints
Training: 6 x 60-min sessions per week including 3–4 hard sessions
Mindset: Feel strong and energetic • Sense of purpose and pride in appearance • Fitness and mental grit integral to personality
Mission Analysis: Requires frequent investments in training, lifestyle planning and vigilance • Optimal health range • Training process builds optimism, self-reliance & grit • Easy to maintain if single or in fitness-related career • Requires careful planning to maintain with young children and sedentary job

GOAL-SETTING TIPS

- Start with a stretch goal – something that excites and scares you.
- Make sure your goal is SMART (Specific, Measurable, Achievable, Relevant, Time-specific).
- Next, pair your stretch goal with a smaller goal. This is your system for turning a 3–5-year ambition into something concrete that changes what you're doing tomorrow.
- Short-term goals have more motivational impact than long-term goals, because they provide quicker feedback on progress, but long-term goals encourage you to test the boundaries of what you're capable of.
- Goals must be challenging, but achievable: if too easy, the goal will feel boring and is unlikely to instigate action; if too difficult, it will be demotivating.
- Feedback enhances the effectiveness of goal-setting, enabling you to adjust your behaviour in order to achieve your goal.
- Specific goals (e.g. running a marathon in under a set time) are more effective than general goals (e.g. getting fitter), because they provide objective criteria to measure your performance against.
- Always go for goal quality over goal quantity.
- When measuring progress towards your goals, using your starting point as the benchmark of comparison is more likely to be motivating for long-term stretch goals.
- Maintaining motivation will likely be determined by external factors (e.g. positive feedback); interactive factors (e.g. a public goal such as fear of public failure) and internal factors (e.g. self-reliance).
- According to Harvard University research, making your goal public and reviewing progress weekly with a friend almost doubles your success rate.
- Use the performance cycle (pages 160–161) to get the best from goal-setting, constantly evaluating your goal so you can adapt your approach, including changes outside your control (e.g. a race being cancelled).
- Before you've even broken a sweat, when setting your own goals, be brutally honest and realistic with what's right for where you are in life.

PLANNING LIKE YOU'VE 10 MINUTES LEFT TO LIVE

To bring the benefits of undergoing mission analysis, war gaming and rehearsal to life, humour me for a minute and consider the following analogy. Imagine your life distilled to a 10-minute shopping sprint in an unknown supermarket containing almost anything you could possibly want and the contents of your basket representing the quality of your life: your experiences, relationships, accomplishments and contributions.

Now pause for a second and reflect on how many times you've found yourself at a real supermarket checkout, staring into a basket containing items you needed, along with some gaps, compromises and impulse buys.

But let's assume you have 24 hours to plan your 10 minutes. What steps will you take to set yourself up for success?

How might you incorporate the process of military analysis, war gaming and rehearsals to shape the next 24 hours' preparation if your life depended on it? Here's how you might prepare.

Mission analysis:
- Create a list to identify all the things you think you want.
- Review your list, reconciling the purpose of each item and whether it's viable to achieve everything when time is so scarce.
- Prioritize each item: what must be removed to preserve space for the essentials?
- What sacrifices are you willing to make to secure the things at the top of your list?

War gaming and rehearsal:
- Research the mission by consulting someone who has done it before, to learn from their experience.
- Use a layout of the store to plan your route, overlaying all items on the map.
- Determine whether 'nice to have' items are collocated with an 'essential' item and therefore can be collected with only marginal effort.
- Secure the help of others in the planning phase, recruiting assistants who know each aisle within the store and can help war game your plan to increase its chance of success.
- Pre-mortem the plan to anticipate potential issues and how they might be mitigated; e.g. how will you react if there's no shopping trolley or a critical item on your list is missing?
- Rehearse the component parts (running with the trolley, stacking items to maximize available space, etc.) and then improve each element, before putting it all together.

It barely requires more than a few moments to appreciate the performance gap between an activity you fall into and a precisely planned and rehearsed operation. Yet, I'm willing to bet despite hundreds of hours of relevant shopping experience you've often found yourself with a basket of unwanted compromises at the end of a hasty shopping trip. A behaviour pattern of stumbling into things unconsciously and confusing hurried activity with effectiveness is familiar to us all. While a shopping trolley missing vegetables and overloaded with celebrity magazines seems inconsequential, a passive approach to life will likely lead to notable gaps and regrets at the end of it. Our capacity is bound by limited resources, whether money, annual holiday or the 168 hours we have every week. Knowing what you want is everything and choosing what to delete is essential. I suspect you'll either love or loathe my approach to this conundrum, but for me it's been a gift that keeps on giving.

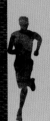

OPTIMIZING YOUR PERSONAL BATTLE RHYTHM

Paratroopers depend on their battle rhythm (see page 79) to thrive in dynamic and hostile environments. Regardless of the mission, it is used to orchestrate activity – daily, weekly and monthly. Its very consistency and dependency is the cornerstone of the regiment's effectiveness.

In my first year outside the regiment, I wrestled hard against balancing work and family commitments. In trying to do everything, be everywhere and retain decision rights on all things, I quickly realized I was on a collision course with burnout, which neither my family, my health nor my colleagues could afford. So, having conducted an effective mission analysis and defined my goals, I concentrated all my effort on optimizing my battle rhythm, so it would provide both the capacity and resilience I needed to thrive in my new operating environment.

TIPS FOR BUILDING YOUR OWN BATTLE RHYTHM

Our lives have a pattern, even if undefined. As these patterns evolve to address changing commitments, we often find ourselves with a collage of legacy activities completely detached from the goals we now pursue. Much of our lives can be codified and to do so preserves the time spent contemplating the same decision every day. Every component of a battle rhythm makes unique contributions to overall efficiency, relieving the frictions of an overburdened schedule. Clarifying our goals and creating and sticking to a personal battle rhythm tunes our focus and reduces stress. Approaching routine things routinely conserves bandwidth to focus attention at critical points and times. A well-refined battle rhythm creates capacity to operate at a sustained level of efficiency for extended periods. A personal battle rhythm includes:

- building and refining practices aligned to the pursuit of your goals;
- refining processes and establishing your own SOPs on a daily and weekly basis;
- creating and preserving the structure of your day;
- establishing healthy sleep/rest routines;
- instituting nutrition plans aligned to your activity levels;
- synchronizing work, personal and family activities and logistics;
- clarifying responsibilities, expectations and decisions with people whom you depend on and who depend on you.

A personal battle rhythm seeks to squeeze the most out of every one of the 168 hours you have in a week as well as ensuring it aligns with your goals. Time, like money, is a scarce resource; while we're able to manage money carefully, we're often prone to squander time wilfully. Committing thought and time to consider how best to achieve a goal is the starting point of every battle rhythm. After this, an optimized personal battle rhythm is built on three components:

1. Prioritization. The mission analysis of all your goals provides the assessment criteria for every activity in your weekly battle rhythm. As illustrated in the shopping trolley analogy, by saying yes to one thing, we're saying no to an infinite number of other things. Whenever you're spending time on something, ask Why am I doing it? What goal does it serve? What happens if I don't do it? By saying yes to this, what am I saying no to? Nothing is better for your battle rhythm than the frequent deployment of 'no' to any activity that is not directly aligned to your goals.

2. Turn routine activities into SOPs. The force multipliers in every battle rhythm are investments made today that yield significantly more free time in the future: automation, delegation and outsourcing are great examples, but it extends way beyond these. Build and refine patterns of behaviour for frequently performed tasks so that they become instinctive in their application and no longer consume your mental energy. Each iteration should end in a better result and consume less time. By making everyday tasks routine, you create the conditions for you to channel your time, energy and talent for maximum impact. You can even scale this process to routine interactions with work colleagues (e.g. team meetings: format, frequency and duration) and family activities (e.g. family meals: planning, preparation and clearing away). Another key element is understanding how much an hour of your time is worth, so you are able to decide whether to do something yourself or pay someone else to do it.

3. Efficiency: Maximize productivity and remove waste. Productivity requires constant vigilance against unproductive and inefficient patterns of behaviour – things that either slow you down or derail you from achieving your goals. While some require little thought to recognize – e.g. funding an hour's surfing on social media with an hour's sleep – some are less obvious. For instance, avoiding time-wasting behaviours (e.g. instead of heading for Starbucks every day, buy a coffee machine), sequencing activities in close proximity to one another (e.g. refuelling your car and getting cash from the ATM at a set time every week) and co-mingling similar tasks (e.g. all computer-based tasks) are all great efficiency drives. Productive behaviours are those things that build momentum in your day: getting up early on the first alarm instead of hitting the snooze button, doing your hardest mental tasks first when your brain is at its best, and listening to audiobooks while training, so you train your mind concurrently with your body.

EXAMPLE BATTLE RHYTHM

On the following pages are some examples of the building blocks I have deployed to establish a more efficient personal battle rhythm. Many are replicable or could serve as inspiration to hunt for your own opportunities to prioritize your time appropriately and maximize your efficiency.

No matter how busy your life, every hour spent optimizing your personal battle rhythm will pay for itself many times over. **A saving of 5 minutes on any daily activity yields 30 hours over the course of a year.** What could be more productive than reclaiming time to pursue your fitness, career and personal goals?

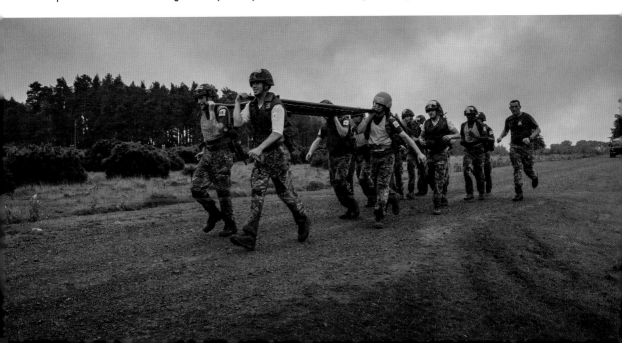

BATTLE RHYTHM

1: PRIORITIZATION

- Schedule all goals at start of year and break down into quarters, to make each more precise and achievable.
- Schedule all annual leave at start of year with 3–5-day buffer for unforeseen events.
- Budget all expenses annually, monthly, weekly to avoid being caught out.
- Budget 168 hours per week (sleep, work, family, hobbies, friends).
- Allocate 1 hour on Friday to plan the next working week so it doesn't play on your mind over the weekend. If in a management role, share it with your team so they have full transparency.
- On Sunday evening review last week against goals, define 3 things to improve/stop doing, and plan the week ahead.
- Treat all hours the same; an hour spent in the gym is the same as an hour spent surfing social media.
- Treat all money the same; your bank account doesn't know the difference between a pound saved on your lunch and a pound saved on your car.
- Determine 3–5 things you need to do but are putting off; allocate set time to complete the most important one and repeat the following day.
- Use shared calendars and actively share with all people who would benefit from knowing what you're up to and ask them to do the same, whether it is a family calendar, a work calendar shared with colleagues or both.

2: ROUTINE ACTIVITIES TO SOPS

- Optimize commute. It should be time and cost efficient.
- Plan meals a week in advance to make sure you support your nutritional needs and have all the ingredients.
- Do all household shopping online. Save weekly lists that correlate to your meal plans.
- Spend 3 hours batch cooking major meals for reheating during the week.
- Pay bills by direct debit. Manage subscriptions to avoid wasting money on something you no longer need.
- Go paper free. Use e-receipts and file everything online.
- Simplify work wardrobe. I only wear dark trousers, black shoes and white shirts. I found a brand that fits well and never give a second thought to what I'm wearing.
- Refine lists of 5–10 cheap/free 2–3-hour family outings or indoor activities to choose from when planning the week.
- Integrate all kids' extra-curricular activities at school or during the week to maximize family time at weekends.
- Establish patterns of time to spend with friends and loved ones to make sure it always happens.
- Build a presentation format/standing agenda for frequent work meetings.
- If in a management role, use 15-min daily stand-up meeting with team. I took this straight from the PARAs. Everyone knows each other's tasks, can request help if needed, and has autonomy for the rest of the day.

3: MINIMIZE WASTEFUL ACTIVITIES

- If you watch TV, consider switching to on-demand or Netflix, so you can watch what you want when you want.
- Remove alerts from phone, laptop, etc. Research suggests it can take up to 15 minutes to recover from distraction when concentrating on a task.
- Delete social media apps to remove temptation to check during the day.
- Browse the Internet for a specific purpose, to avoid wasting time on things that are interesting but unimportant.
- To prevent sleep disruption, avoid caffeine after 2pm and leave phone outside bedroom.
- Avoid eating 3 hours before bed, so all your food is digested properly.
- Avoid too much alcohol – it kills your time, money and judgement.
- Remove visibility status on messaging apps, so you can respond when convenient.
- Block work online calendar at least 1 week in advance, to avoid people bulldozing your time at short notice.
- Get your clothes and lunch ready the night before to maximize sleep and save time.
- If possible work from home a couple of days per week to avoid time spent commuting.
- Buy a coffee machine for the office to avoid going out for coffee. Buying coffee is at least a 20-minute task.
- De-clutter to avoid losing hours looking for stuff.

4: MAXIMIZE PRODUCTIVE ACTIVITIES

- Get up early, so you're alert. If you start the day in a rush, it's often impossible to recover from it.
- Train in dead time when family are sleeping, ideally before work.
- Integrate training into commute to get double benefit.
- Train with close friends, making training a social activity and building an additional level of accountability.
- Listen to audiobooks/podcasts while training, to train mind and body simultaneously. I find this only works for light-effort cardio sessions, but still consume 20 books a year this way.
- Use public transport, so you can read, watch Ted talks, respond to emails, catch up with friends, etc., while concurrently saving money on owning a second car.
- Go to bed and wake up at same time every day. This helps build your circadian rhythm, made even more effective if you train outside in daylight first thing.
- Make all major and financial decisions in the morning, when you're at your most vigilant.
- Plan all meetings and calls in advance, including the objectives, responsibilities and follow-up timelines.
- Use associative triggers to make you more effective. I always have a coffee while reviewing my plan for the day, so when my body smells coffee it knows it's planning time.
- Turn off your work phone at 7pm and don't check it before leaving the house the next day, to avoid thinking about work during family time.

THE BRUNEVAL RAID – OPERATION *BITING*

Overcoming fear and anxiety through preparation and rehearsal

In 1942, RAF bombers were incurring heavy losses. These were caused by advances in German radar technology, which was increasingly able to locate RAF aircraft at a distance. British aircraft would then be intercepted by German fighters and destroyed before they could carry out their mission. British scientists were eager to understand German advances in order to create countermeasures to neutralize their effect and simultaneously advance the Allies' own radar systems. A German radar station located on the coast at Bruneval, in northern France, was identified as a suitable site to capture both the equipment and the operators for interrogation. However, it was concluded that an amphibious operation was likely to incur heavy casualties due to the proximity of local reinforcements and naval patrol boats. Therefore, the only solution was an airborne raid.

Planning

Operation *Biting* fell to C Company, 2 PARA, commanded by Major John Frost. Major Frost's plan was for a night-time airborne insertion of 130 men, who would then be extracted after the raid by naval landing craft. However, the PARAs faced several significant challenges before they even left England. C Company had only just been formed and fewer than half its men were parachute-trained, with even fewer being able to swim – which was necessary for them to reach the landing craft. Parachuting was in its infancy and none of the RAF pilots assigned to the mission had conducted a drop. Information on the radar station was scant and little was known about the German guard strength or the speed and strength of local German Army reserves. This would be the first operational descent for the PARAs, and not only would the safety of the RAF bombers depend on the mission being a success, but so too would the future of the Parachute Regiment.

Preparation

C Company commenced a consolidated period of training and rehearsal for the raid, continually improving their plan with the RAF and Royal Navy units supporting them. Major Frost's first challenge was to ensure that no soldier was fazed by either the insertion or the extraction, so mastering swimming and parachuting was their first goal. Secondly, the company built a scale model of the radar station on the bank of a Scottish loch and practised each aspect of the plan separately: the insertion, the attack, the dismantling of the radar equipment, the extraction of the equipment and operators to the boat meeting point and the extraction by landing craft. Finally, C Company put all of the parts of the plan together and drilled it until everyone knew their part perfectly. In parallel the Royal Navy and RAF analysed the environmental factors that would best ensure success – identifying that a raid in late February would give C Company the perfect combination of clear skies, high tide and a long period of darkness to conduct their mission.

Execution

On the evening of 27 February 1942, Operation *Biting* was launched and was a complete success. C Company suffered only a few casualties during the raid and captured both the radar equipment and operators, which ultimately proved the capability of airborne forces and led to the RAF developing effective countermeasures, saving a countless number of lives.

Re-evaluate the plan and the result

The Bruneval raid is still widely acknowledged as a brilliantly executed airborne operation, and I believe there are many lessons from it that can be transferred into any highly stressed performance setting. By analysing the mission, Major Frost was able to break the task down into proximate goals (learning to swim, breaking down radar, etc). Sequentially tackling each component part and then combining them all together once mastered prevented C Company from being overwhelmed by the enormity of their task. By isolating the company for training, Frost was able to remove any external pressure and focus everyone on the task at hand rather than on the consequences of failure. By integrating the RAF and Royal Navy into his planning process, he was able to use their expertise to conduct specific PARA and amphibious training, as well as to identify the ideal timing for the raid – leaving C Company to focus on getting the ground plan right.

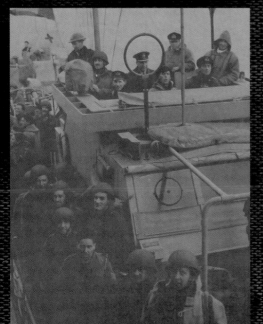

Major Frost and the men of 2 PARA after the raid.

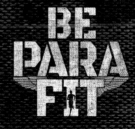

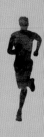

FINDING YOUR OWN P COMPANY

The term 'paratrooper' is incongruent with half-measures. At the outset my mantra was to pick a stretch goal that intimidates and excites you. Do not be constrained by the standards or even the examples in this book – find your own P Company. **A fitness programme built on weight loss is temporary. A fitness programme based on continually pushing your own performance frontiers is a learning experience, not a losing experience.** If the goal you choose is achievable without having to lay stable foundations in your sleeping patterns, your nutrition and your mobility, you're thinking too small. The more audacious the goal, the more we must innovate across the system to achieve it, testing all your physical resources and invading your psychology – just like paratrooper selection.

Overruling comfort and certainty, and demanding things of your mind and body that others consider reckless, builds confidence in your ability to intelligently adapt to meet changing needs. This is critical for success, not just on the battlefield but in all aspects of life. Whether it's joining the Parachute Regiment or crossing the finish line on something that's right for you, I believe the transformation and experience will be the same, regardless of how long it takes you to you achieve it: a mind and body that's 'ready for anything'.

The perfect training plan will be unique to your goal and circumstances, which will change frequently and require constant adjustment, but I can share some enduring principles that have worked for me.

COMPETITION

If your goal isn't P Company, my advice is to choose a progressive ladder of competition; there's no better driver of performance and innovation. A training cycle rich in competition facilitates growth by continually processing and reviewing performance in test conditions. Just like P Company, competition is less about what you get from it and the end of the race, than what you can give and how it changes you in the process. The goal isn't merely the podium or even the time, but the mentality of being prepared physically and psychologically. The blend of anticipation, excitement and fear competition creates is the best proxy I've found for embarking on a well-planned and rehearsed military mission. There's a 'tribalness' to competition even in individual sports like ultra-marathon running, which transcends gender, age, culture and postcode. The more intense the task and personal challenge, the stronger the connection between you and other competitors. Even in the most adversarial of sports there is a mutual respect, forged from shared hardships. Just like paratrooper selection, surrounding yourself with people who are all pushing themselves to be the best version of themselves is a sure-fire formula to success.

MENTAL PREPARATION: ANTICIPATE, ALIGN AND ADAPT

Any stretch goal, requiring months of focused planning and disciplined execution, is funded by sacrifices and discipline. To commit to a stretch goal demands a conscious understanding about the pain, discomfort and personal concessions you are willing to endure to make it possible. It requires both research and a plan. As discussed above, you'll need to assess your mission and make some tough decisions on activities that aren't aligned to your goals. The critical success factor, however, will be building a support network across work, family and friends to make it possible, or else you'll find yourself constantly battling with those you care the most about in the pursuit of your goal. All parties need to know the rules of engagement, so your relationships complement rather than compete with your goal.

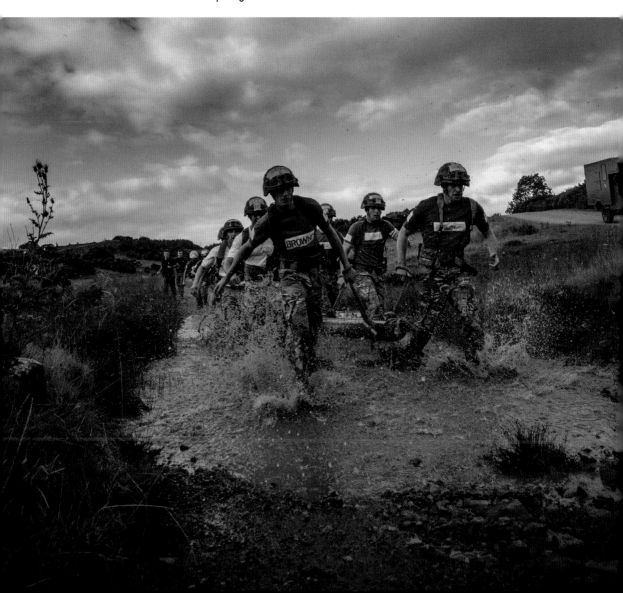

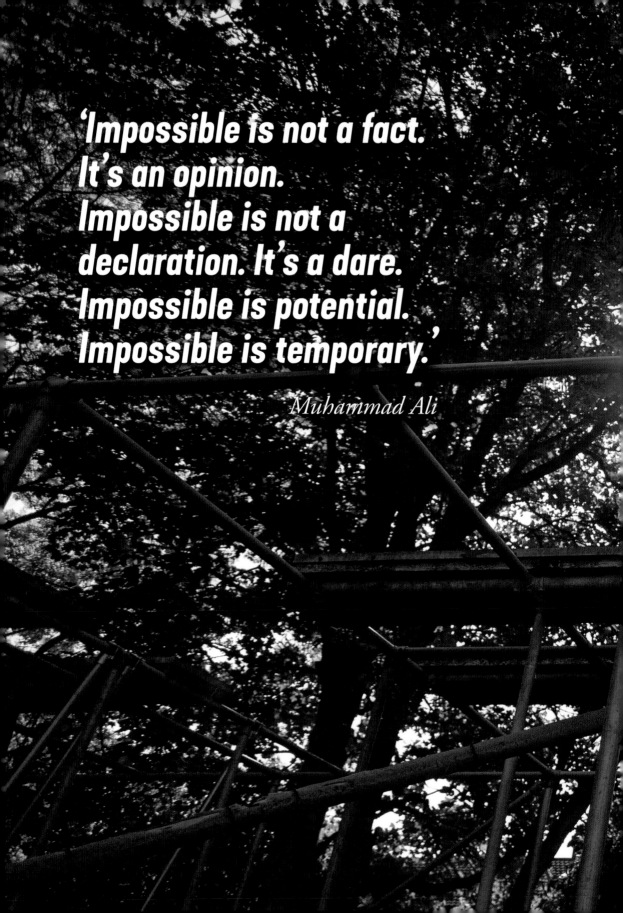

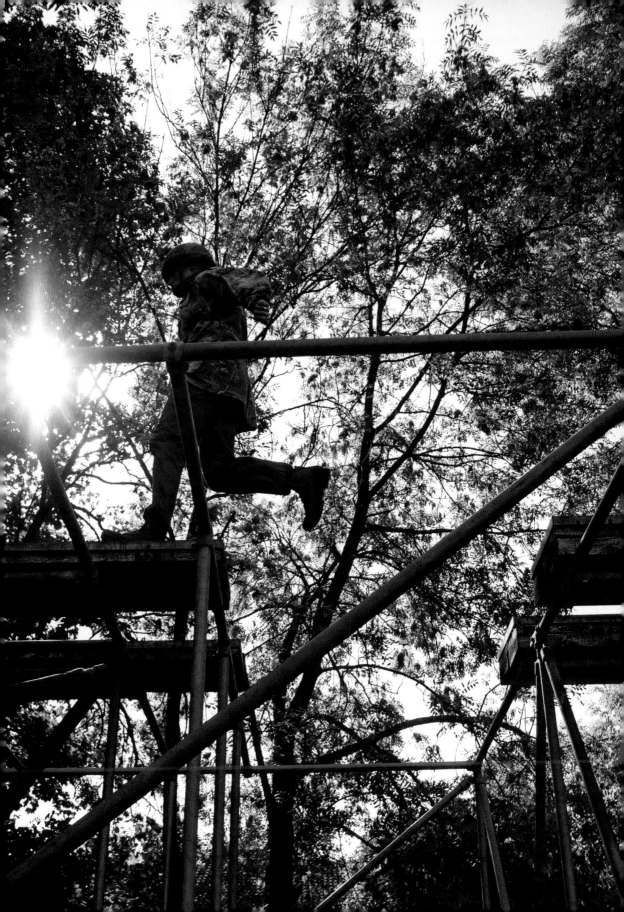

LEARNING FROM FAILURE

Having created and committed to a stretch goal, it might be surprising to hear that the next thing you need to do is to accept that failure is a vital source of feedback en route to success. All seasoned paratroopers know no plan survives contact with the enemy. The same will be true for your plan: you might find it doesn't work out as you had anticipated and will need regular modification. Sustained performance belongs to those that remain agile and evolve, through a mix of vision, creativity and measurement. We study military failures, not just successes, because failure creates the burning platform often needed to ignite meaningful change.

AFTER ACTION REVIEW

By ignoring lessons of failure in the short term, you invite bigger losses in the long term. In the PARAs we recognize this and undertake an after action review (AAR) after every mission. The AAR is a forum where all parts of the mission, not just the result, are discussed so we can refine future missions. The underlying principle of the AAR is that the learning advantage of adapting outweighs the reputational consequences of drawing attention to an issue.

In the PARAs our lives depend on candour, a quality all too often lacking in most other organizations. Rank is left outside the room and feedback is valued on its merits and its rigour. Through the AAR we are able to get to the best outcome for future missions. It's a process that is directly transferable to the cycle of performance in any domain, but especially training and competition.

If something goes wrong with your training or in a competition conduct your own AAR. Be brutally honest with yourself and if there are others you can ask for feedback do. Don't shy away from acknowledging what went wrong and how. Next time you will not repeat the same mistakes and you will excel because of it.

THE PERFORMANCE CYCLE

The only thing more important than selecting a clear and unambiguous training goal is your philosophy to it. What links elite military units, high-performing corporate teams and world-class athletes is an approach to excellence and, specifically, goals. The highest achievers have the clearest, most concise goals and timetables for achievement. The performance cycle is a system, aligned to proactively innovate and push your frontiers, comprising four key steps:

1. Create a plan with a clear timetable.
2. Execute the plan.
3. Re-evaluate the plan and improve it.
4. Take responsibility for results, good and bad.

The perfect training plan is the culmination of a journey towards mastery, not the starting point. This means steps 2 and 3 require the most focus. As outlined above, the process calls for us to embrace failure and learn from it. Be agile. The shorter the cycle between execution, evaluation and improvement iterations – the better. If you're not embarrassed by your first results you have procrastinated too much with your first plan.

If adopted and refined, the performance cycle can be applied to every type of goal. It is less about the view from the summit of one of these challenges, than the attitude it fosters getting there: a will to win and an unwavering determination in the face of adversity. This will mean that step 4 is never the end of your fitness journey; instead, you simply set new challenges and continuously work your way through the performance cycle.

What follows are some challenges I believe are worth pursuing, to get you going; goals of sufficient size that they require multi-phase cycles of plan, execution and re-evaluation. To keep things interesting, I've included my own current training goal last. So, if we ever meet, or you happen to be called Eliza, Nellie, Bea or Tess McGrath – feel free to call me out if it remains unfinished business...

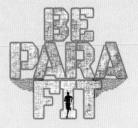

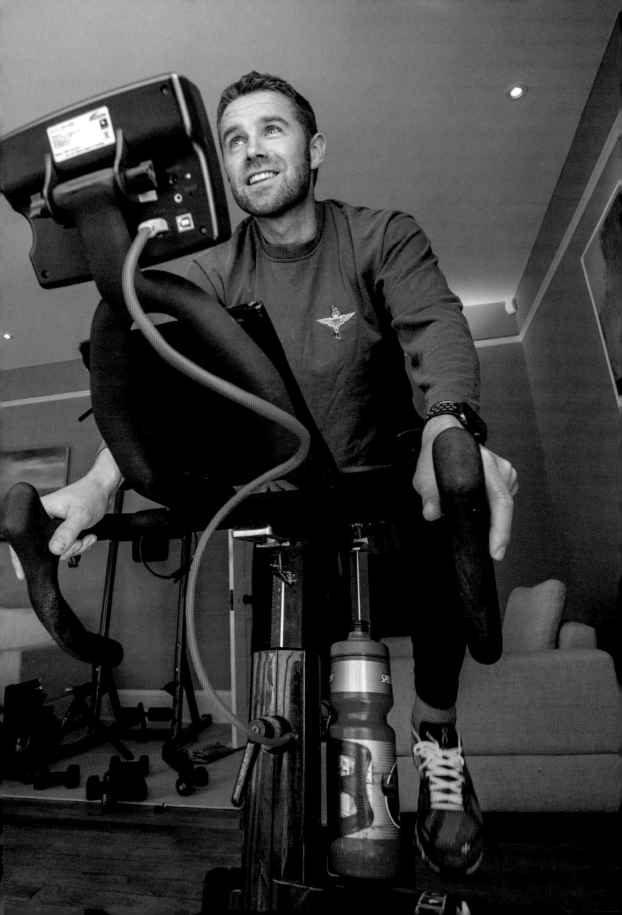

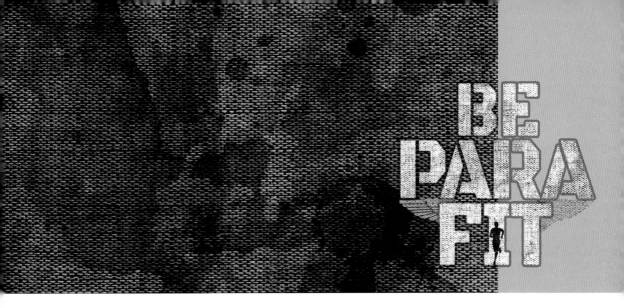

Chapter 7

CHALLENGES

While I have arranged these challenges in ascending order of difficulty, confronting any competition to achieve a personal best will test your mental and physical resolve. The fitter you get, the harder you must work to ascend to new heights. It would be possible to enter all bar the final challenge without first proving your mettle on some form of gateway challenge, but I would strongly advise against this. Running with others affects your pace; it is simply impossible not to adjust your pace when someone either passes you or is within a couple of purposeful strides. I believe the best way to improve your running is through road-running races, which are relatively cheap and frequent, making them accessible to most people who live near a medium-sized town. The ideal starting point is 'The Park Run', a free 5km race that takes place every week in the parks of most major towns and cities. So, regardless of how confident you may feel tackling either a marathon or ultra-marathon immediately, there are two reasons why you should rethink this. First, you won't have the race experience to do your fitness justice – your pace and final result will be cannibalized by trying to keep up with fitter runners. Second, achieving the minimum aptitude standard is incongruent with the PARA ethos; walking over the line of your first marathon may earn you a t-shirt but it won't come with the physical mettle or mindset we're striving for. The benchmark is a 1hr 40min half-marathon (1hr 50min for females) before tackling longer challenges; otherwise you risk injury, not finishing or being so embarrassed with your result it deters you from doing another.

THE HALF-MARATHON: FIGHTING FIT STANDARD

The half-marathon is an event that blends long distance with speed. Regardless of your fitness and running ability, it provides a great challenge and training goal. Unlike longer events, both the time required and running routes for half-marathon training are easier to find, which is why I believe it is within the grasp of most recreational runners and anyone comfortable on the Fighting Fit programme.

What I really like about half-marathons is that you get such a broad spectrum of runners taking part; depending on the profile of the event you can have everyone from Olympic athletes to people wearing deep-sea diver costumes. You can guarantee that you won't come last. Having already flagged the importance of securing the support of your friends and family, the half-marathon is a perfect platform for them to both see the fruits of all your hard training and share in your success. The larger events have carnival-like atmospheres, motivating music and race routes lined with supporters cheering you on.

THE MARATHON: FIGHTING FIT TO PARATROOPER STANDARD

In the half-marathon, the challenge is roughly 80% physical and 20% mental, but in the marathon these percentages are reversed. The distance of the marathon, both for training and race day, makes it more than twice as difficult. Running a marathon requires concerted training effort and significantly longer runs in preparation for race day. Expect halfway in the mental race to be around the 20-mile point and you won't be far wrong. But, while the marathon may be more than twice as difficult as the half, the sense of achievement is incomparable. In Chapter 1, I described the role of P Company in teaching prospective PARAs what they're capable of – this is exactly what you'll get from your first marathon. You don't need to be of Paratrooper-level fitness standards to tackle your first marathon, but you should have at least reached the Paratrooper programme and be capable of running 16km/10 miles in under 75 minutes (male) or 85 minutes (female). You will need to supplement your training with a specific marathon programme; 12 weeks should be ample. I'd advocate using an online programme from a reputable fitness magazine, or a virtual coach if you're looking for something tailored to you.

ROAD-RACING TIPS

On the basis that this may be your first road race ever or for some time, here are some things that should help you in your preparations.

Train hard, fight easy

You should never do anything in competition that you haven't first honed in training, but there's one caveat – above half-marathon, you don't need to do the full distance. Covering 80% of race distance about a month beforehand is the sweet spot; you'll be at peak fitness but with sufficient time before your race to be fully recovered. Like any rehearsal, this longer race is more about mental preparation than physical. During the race, you will fight a constant battle against giving up – you need to get a taste of this in training so you're mentally equipped to push through it in the heat of the moment. Remember: the real prize is the grit formed in training and on race day, not the medal.

Water and food stations

Remaining hydrated during any race over 10km/6 miles is critical, but food becomes equally important in marathons since your body will deplete its carbohydrate stores after roughly two hours of continuous exercise. Fuel stations are commonplace in road races over 5km/3 miles, but you'll need to incorporate eating and drinking into your training runs as it takes some getting used to. As with many things in things in life, less is more. Try to consume small amounts of food, water and electrolytes at every station to replenish salt lost through sweating. Too much water vs isotonic and you'll be prone to cramping; too much electrolytes and you'll feel thirsty, tired and may have trouble concentrating. I typically take an energy gel every 45 minutes and alternate between water and isotonic drinks.

Mile markers

Having drummed in the importance of breaking down a challenge into smaller goals, in an organized race much of this is done for you with distance markers. Use these markers to your advantage as your short-term focus, but always keep one eye on the finish line. Before you start, have a plan for your desired time, then use that time to work out when you need to be at each marker. This will keep you on track and maintain your focus throughout the race.

Massed starts

Unless you are an elite runner, massed starts are a necessary evil and they will slow you down a little. You need to prepare for this and factor it into your planning. Plan on not being able to run at your chosen pace for at least the first mile; the more people running the race the greater the friction, but it's normally made up for by more spectators cheering you on. What's important is that you anticipate being behind when you get to your first couple of checkpoints, and you have the chance to think about how you intend to claw your time back without ruining your race by going too quickly when the path clears ahead of you.

Relax

On the battlefield, much of what happens to us is outside of our control. But in the Parachute Regiment what distinguishes us is how we thrive in chaos. Inevitably, on your first race things won't go to plan, but provided you see the whole thing in the wider context of tackling the most significant fitness challenge of your life, it is possible to win the war even if the battle leaves scar tissue. Define success as feeling motivated to do another race, not breaking the course record.

Share your success

Training for any significant fitness race such as a half- or full marathon can put an incredible strain on your relationships. Do not be shy in showing your appreciation to all who have helped you find the time and motivation to attempt this race. Aside from being the right thing to do, it will maintain their commitment in the future. Why not treat them all at the end to say 'thank you' for their support? Nothing will erode your future training opportunities more than complaining about your performance to those who sacrificed things to support you in your preparation – they won't make the same mistake again. Tell them what a marvellous experience it was – especially if it wasn't.

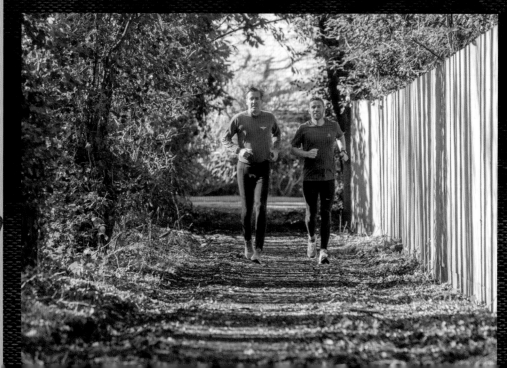

THE PARAS' 10: FIGHTING FIT TO PARATROOPER STANDARD

The PARAs' 10 is based on the P Company 10-miler described in Chapter 1. The 10-miler is a core paratrooper test, designed to simulate the move between the parachute drop zone and our objective. The 35lb Bergen simulates a paratrooper's fighting order (the ammunition and equipment carried into battle). As well as being a P Company test event, which all volunteers must pass, it is a weekly feature in PARA battalion life. However, what makes the PARAs' 10 unique as an endurance event is that you effectively do a paratrooper's 10-miler in its entirety – 35lb Bergen, military boots, same route and same time. The cut-off time is 1 hour 50 minutes. The only thing that differs from the real paratrooper test is the lack of weapons (put in an extra 10lb if you want), but by tackling it you will get a real sense of whether you have what it takes to pass a PARA test. However, first a word of caution: this is the easy bit, for what follows the 10-miler on the real battlefield is a fight for your life.

The race is staged in September so the weather is normally quite mild, but the Catterick weather has been known to be changeable. The route is more hilly than mountainous, but it is enclosed entirely within the Catterick military training area, making it much more scenic and exposed than most road runs. However, there are water and first aid stations at the 4- and 8-mile points.

When I commanded P Company, I tackled the 10-miler with monotonous regularity, completing it under test conditions with a course at least every fortnight. I believe TAB-ing (Tactical Advance to Battle) is picked up easily – all you need is a good base level of fitness, well-fitted boots and a relatively comfy Bergen. The trick is to traverse the ground as efficiently as possible; while some would be capable of running the whole route, your best bet is to stride up the hills and maintain a steady jog on all the flats and the downhill sections. As with any route of moderate distance, it is vital that you maintain your energy and hydration levels.

The added annoyance of heavy boots and an equipment-laden Bergen gives the race a PARA authenticity – one that you will only enjoy after the event, when you're telling your mates about your achievement.

SPARTAN ADVENTURE RACE: FIGHTING FIT TO PARATROOPER STANDARD

Founded in 300 AD and revived in 2007, Spartan is now an international phenomenon that occurs in over 42 countries. A combination of grit and fitness, Spartan is a series of obstacle challenges rather than just a race. Spartan events cater for a broad range of abilities and pain thresholds, including the Spartan Sprint (3 miles and 20 obstacles), suitable for someone starting the Fighting Fit programme; the Spartan Super (8 miles and 25 obstacles), suitable for someone comfortable on the Fighting Fit programme; the Spartan Beast (13 miles and 30 obstacles), suitable for someone comfortable on the Paratrooper programme; and the Ultra Beast (26 miles and 60 obstacles), suitable for someone on the Paratrooper/P Company programme, with some additional marathon training.

The obstacles are designed to intimidate; most share a military assault course heritage, requiring strength, agility and muscular endurance in spades. They test functional fitness and grit concurrently, by pushing competitors to breaking point. Obstacle formats vary from race to race, making surprise a key ingredient of every Spartan experience. Favourites include mud crawling, fire runs, heavy object carries, ice water submersions, tyre flips, rope climbs and tractor pulls. Spartan has managed to deliver a safe experience which cuts across modern-day health and safety mollycoddling. Mild hypothermia, grazed

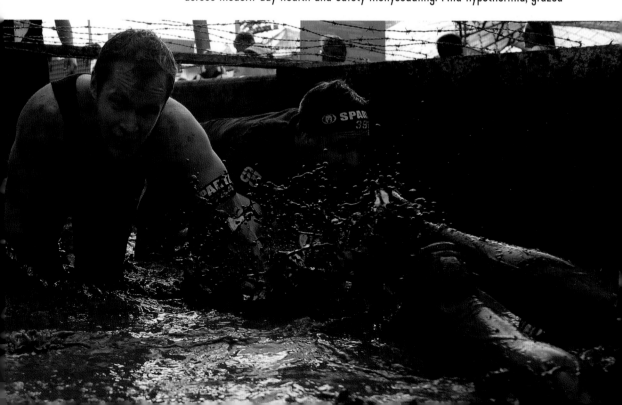

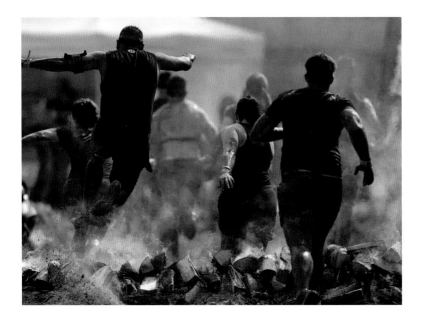

knees and black-and-blue limbs are par for the course, which makes Spartan both deeply unpleasant and retrospectively enjoyable. With modern-day pampering firmly in its crosshair, Spartan accepts children over four into abridged circuits that remain true to their philosophy. But as the saying goes – if you're going to be a bear, be a grizzly, so don't settle for anything less than the 26-mile 100-obstacle Ultra Beast!

This unique cocktail of challenge attracts over 1 million entrants annually. For Spartans, like Paratroopers, the game always changes after the starter pistol has been fired. While military set pieces are finessed and rehearsed, it's unlikely they'll play out that way. The hazard and uncertainty of arduous training is what helps the warrior thrive at their lowest ebb – Spartan agree and have cut their cloth accordingly:

> Spartan is more than a race; it's a way of life. We believe that you can't have a strong body without a strong mind, that you can't grow without pressure, that obstacles help shift our frame of reference and make us more resilient. We believe that signing up for a race holds us accountable and keeps us motivated to train harder and eat healthier.*

I would equate the gulf between preparing for a road-running race vs Spartan, to the difference between preparing for a bar room brawl vs the lead role in the Bolshoi ballet.

* www.spartan.com

ULTRA-MARATHONS: PARATROOPER STANDARD +

While the marathon (26.2 miles/42.2km) was born when Pheidippides ran from the Battle of Marathon to Athens to report victory in 490 BC, the origin of the ultra-marathon is less clear and its distance less precise. 'Ultra-marathon' is the term used to describe any race exceeding marathon distance, but at its heart, 'ultra' describes a competition against yourself. Runners confront the unknown doubt and difficulty of an extreme challenge, in the pursuit of an intangible prize – the joy of completion.

Ultras have experienced viral growth in the last decade, quenching the growing thirst for more gruelling mental and physical challenges of the running community. Well within the grasp of an experienced runner who has completed a marathon in under 4 hours, ultras forge character in all who endure them. The uncourageous don't try and the weak give in. While they share the same base name, the grit and camaraderie experienced on an

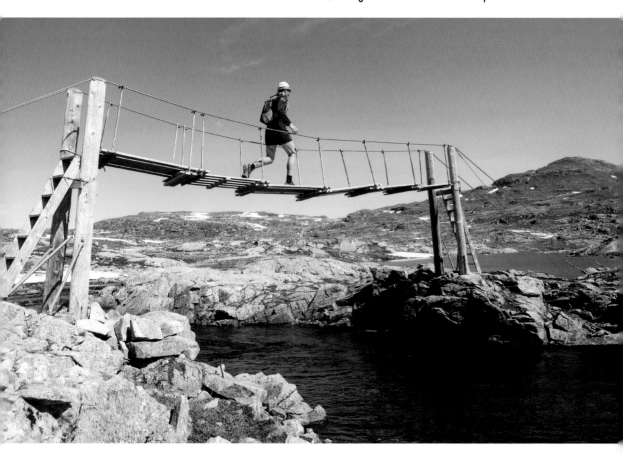

ultra stretch far beyond a standard marathon. In ultras there's not only more distance to cover, but fewer people, fewer water stations and fewer mile markers. Most are off-road, requiring runners to carry both food and safety equipment. Many include significant undulation, are often overnight and take in excess of 24 hours. The International Trail Running Association (ITRA) grade all trail runs over 25km in terms of difficulty, with 1 being the easiest and 6 being the hardest (in excess of 210km). My advice is to use the ITRA scale to guide you; start with a flat 50km race (2 ITRA points) and work upwards. If the marathon is 80% mental, 20% physical, then I'd suggest a 5-point ITRA ultra is 95% mental and a 6-pointer is at least 99% mental. I have taken to using climbing poles to help negotiate 5 ITRA pointers and above, to help preserve my legs for the duration, but the truth is that everything hurts anyway.

Ultras are typically two to three times more expensive to enter than road marathons because they need to cater for emergency medical cover in remote locations. Many involve very early starts and late finishes, with camping not only your most convenient means of accommodation but often included in the entry fee.

On your first race your objective is to reach the finish line uninjured and undeterred from doing another about a week later, but expect some jeopardy along the way. There is nothing quite like the feeling of being utterly exhausted and knowing you're not even halfway around. Expect to rationalize giving up as the most responsible thing to do; all manner of justifications to stop will not only seem plausible for your safety but the only available option. Personally, I enjoy these mental challenges, particularly the prompt they ignite to tap into a well of mental grit that rarely gets the opportunity to surface. Yep, I miss the PARAs. Diarrhoea, vomiting and cramp are par for the course, but soon pass and only make the experience all the more memorable and rewarding with hindsight. Pain disappears on the finish line, and the desire to do another returns after a big plate of warm food and a good night's sleep.

Your first 4-point ITRA ultra will require sustained training effort and significant sacrifices if you complete it running rather than walking. Success demands the full suite of mission analysis and the broader planning process before you even consider your training programme. Once you're convinced it's a viable option, an online running programme from a reputable fitness magazine will set you off in the right direction, but your best bet to achieving a decent result on your first race is with a good virtual coach as described in Chapter 5.

ULTRA-TRAIL MONT BLANC (UTMB)
CHAMONIX, FRANCE: PARATROOPER STANDARD ++

Completing the UTMB is the most coveted prize in ultra-marathon running. Founded in 2002 by nine friends, the UTMB series has since evolved to a portfolio of races from 56km to 290km, of which UTMB is considered the pinnacle. Held annually in the last week of August/first week of September, the challenge beckons 2,300 runners from 92 countries. All runners compete independently along a well-marked route, carrying packs of 3–5kg, including mandatory safety equipment and enough food/water for each stage.

The route traverses Mont Blanc (4,810m), covering 171km of alpine trails through France, Italy and Switzerland. A cumulative ascent of 10,000 meters, extreme climate volatility (-10 to +30 deg C) and a 46-hour cut off justifiably make it the mecca of ultra-trail running. Males and females compete across seven age categories. But it's a race brimming with solidarity: elite and amateur runners share the same start and finish, and with no prize money even for first place, winning is its own reward. The precise race route changes each year, meaning there is no enduring course record. Subject to conditions, elite male runners power home in around 19 hours, with elite females closer to 25 hours. Notwithstanding the scale of the UTMB challenge, the majority of runners are amateurs who complete the course in 30–45 hours. Less than a third drop out either through injury or exhaustion.

Demand for places outstrips supply every year, with four applicants for every place. For safety the race has stringent entrance criteria – this is not a race for have-a-go heroes. All runners must demonstrate their preparedness by first accruing points from a maximum of three global qualifying races within two years of the race. The qualification process and evaluation of feeder races is managed by ITRA. All entrants require 15 ITRA points from three races. A draw is then held to allocate places to runners with sufficient points. For those who want to be certain of a place at the start line, a number of charitable donation places are available, but no latitude is given on the qualifying points. As genuinely elite training goals go, I believe UTMB is the sweet spot – a rare opportunity to compete side by side with the pinnacle of a sport. Subject to you being willing to commit to 10 hours per week of purposeful training for two to three years, reinforced with a surge of 12–16hr weeks in the few months prior to the race, UTMB is a summit you can realistically scale.

Just like the Parachute Regiment, UTMB cares little where you're from – only that you have demonstrated the mental and physical mettle to cross the line of departure surrounded by people who share the same philosophy. Like P Company, it intimidates all who seek to complete it, but ignore the 15 ITRA points for a second, because all will be for nought without a sense of optimism, self-reliance and grit. To be ready for UTMB, you need to be 'ready for anything'. See you there?

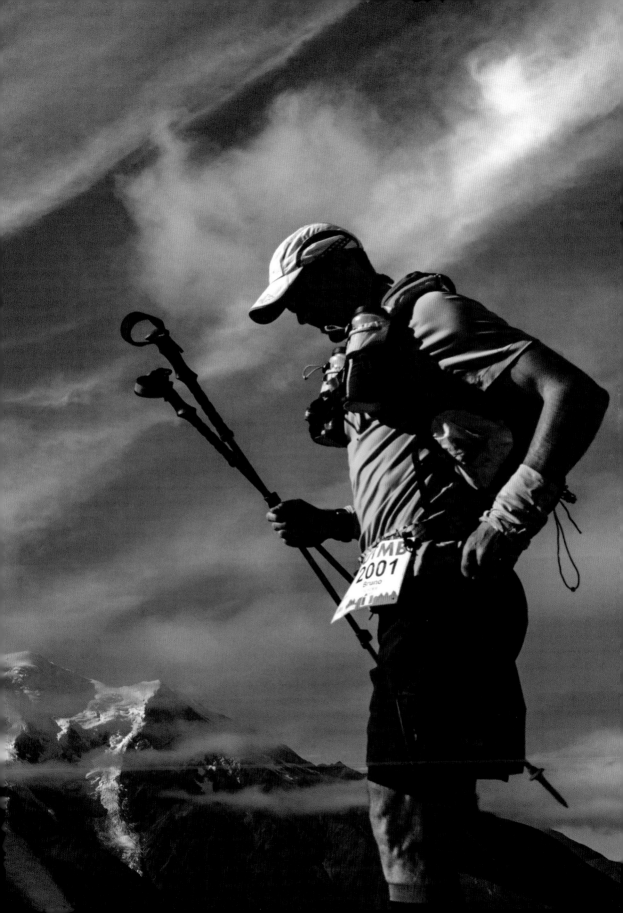

GOAL PLAN

MY SAMPLE STRETCH GOAL PLAN

Complete Ultra-Trail Mont Blanc in Chamonix in 12–18 months' time

Why: Pinnacle of ultra-running in stunning setting. Opportunity to meet like-minded people. Race, qualification and training will test my mental and physical resolve and push my personal boundaries. Preparation will force me to be creative with training, e.g. absence of hills and finding time. Living by my values – example to family, friends and colleagues.

Context: Training time limited to weekends, pre-work and post work. Training competing with family commitments, book-writing schedule and other commitments such as sports coaching on a Saturday morning. Also UTMB takes place during school term time so unable to combine with family holiday.

Outline plan: Qualify this year, take part next year. Qualification process spread out over the year broken down into quarters: select qualifying races in Q1. Use Q1 to build up aerobic base, complete first race in Q2, second race in Q3 and third in Q4.

Whose support is crucial:

- Annie (wife) – needs to be happy with time and financial costs.
- Employer – I will require leave for all qualifying events.

Whose support/advice can help:

- Vlad (coach) – structures training programme to increase likelihood of success.
- Roger (local support) – lives in Chamonix and previously completed UTMB so can provide local advice and support regarding qualification, prep and execution.

Potential Obstacles

1. Injury in lead up to event
2. Not enough points to qualify
3. Injury on UTMB
4. Work commitment
5. Family commitment
6. Loss of Annie's support
7. Inadequate hill training
8. Unsuccessful in race ballot

Potential Root Causes of Obstacles

1. Over-training
2. Unable to complete qualifying race
3. Accident during race
4. Poor planning on my part
5. Family emergency
6. Allow training to creep into family time
7. Lack of hill terrain near home
8. Race oversubscribed

Solutions

1. Disciplined in training and with stretching. Seek physio support as soon as any niggles arise. Use bike to supplement aerobic volume.
2. Identify 4th race in December as potential back up.
3. Ensure medical insurance cover is in place for the race.
4. Forewarn boss and team, forecast and address any potential issues early.
5. Plan ahead and forewarn. Ensure travel insurance in place. Family emergency will always take precedence.
6. Be disciplined in terms of early morning training. Support Annie in identifying her own UTMB/ stretch goal equivalent.
7. Integrate stairs into training every week. Use underground station stairs during daily run commute to work.
8. Consider charity donation option to bypass ballot.

MISSION ESSENTIAL TASKS

MISSION ESSENTIAL TASK 1:
1st QUALIFYING RACE (100KM)
Timeline May
Time Commitments required 12 weeks' training with 10–12 hours per week. 8 hours' sleep per night. 1 day annual leave for travel to race
Already Scheduled Commitments: School half-term holiday: 1 week in February. Business trip: 2 weeks in April
Costs: Race entry £50

MISSION ESSENTIAL TASK 2:
2nd QUALIFYING RACE (100KM)
Timeline September
Time Commitments 12 weeks' training with 10–12 hours per week. 8 hours' sleep per night. 1 day annual leave for travel to race
Already Scheduled Commitments: School summer holidays: 6 weeks in June/July
Costs: Race entry £50

MISSION ESSENTIAL TASK 3:
3rd QUALIFYING RACE (100KM)
Timeline November
Time Commitments 12 weeks' training with 10–12 hours per week. 8 hours' sleep per night. 1 day annual leave for travel to race
Already Scheduled Commitments: Family visit: 2 weeks in November
Costs: Race entry £50

MISSION ESSENTIAL TASK 4:
UTMB ENTRY BALLOT
Timeline 31 December
Time Commitments 1 hour
Costs: Race entry £200

MISSION ESSENTIAL TASK 5:
ARRIVE FIT FOR UTMB
Timeline August
Time Commitments 36 weeks' training with 12–15 hours per week. 3 days' leave for travel and event
Costs: 20 months' coaching plus travel and accommodation: £1,500

TOTAL:
Time Commitments 6 days' annual leave. 10–15 hours average training per week to be built up incrementally to reduce impact on family and work
Costs: £1,850

IMMEDIATE ACTION:
- Secure work and family support for plan outlined above
- Use coach to identify best qualifying races
- Enter first race
- Begin coaching/training
- Reassess plan after first race and after all other qualifying races

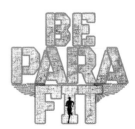

ACKNOWLEDGEMENTS

I owe a tremendous debt of gratitude to all who made *Be Para Fit* a reality:

My girls – Annie, Eliza, Nellie, Bea & Tess.

My editor Kate Moore, Gemma Gardner, Marcus Cowper and many others at Bloomsbury. Matt Timbers, for the excellent images, and Neil Jamieson.

Lieutenant General James Bashall, Charles Heath-Saunders, and the P Company staff and students for their support throughout the project.

My parents, Frank and Emma, for their unconditional love and encouragement and for instilling a belief that everything is possible.

And finally, Winston Churchill, for forming the regiment that inspired this book. In 7 words he captures what took me 40,000:

'I never worry about action, only inaction.' – Winston Churchill

SUPPORT OUR PARAS

SUPPORT OUR PARAS is a charity which supports The Parachute Regiment through the welfare of serving soldiers and families and those affected by recent operations, and through the maintenance of its regimental efficiency, ethos, spirit and heritage. SUPPORT OUR PARAS is the trading name of The Parachute Regiment Charity Ltd, registered as Charity No 1131977 and at Companies House No 07005997.

For more information about the charity, or to find out how you can support us, please visit supportourparas.org or find us on Facebook, Twitter or Instagram @supportourparas

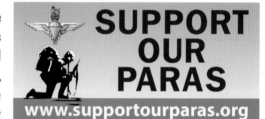

SUPPORT OUR PARAS
www.supportourparas.org
RCN 1131977

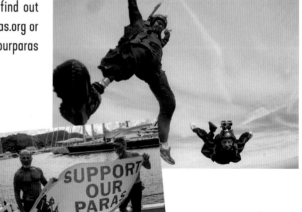